# EXAMINATION MEDICINE

# EXAMINATION MEDICINE

## A Guide to Physician Training

### SECOND EDITION

## Nicholas J. Talley

MB BS, PhD, FRACP, FACP, FACG, FAF PHM

*Associate Professor of Medicine*
*Mayo Medical School*
and
*Consultant*
*Division of Gastroenterology and Internal Medicine*
*Mayo Clinic*
*Rochester, Minnesota, USA*

## Simon O'Connor

BS, MB, FRACP, DDU

*Consultant Cardiologist*
*Royal Canberra Hospital*
*Australia*

**BLACKWELL**
**SCIENTIFIC PUBLICATIONS**
OXFORD LONDON EDINBURGH

First published 1986
Reprinted 1986
Revised 1988
Reprinted 1990
Second Edition 1991

MacLennan & Petty Pty Limited
80 Reserve Road, Artarmon NSW 2064, Australia
© 1991 MacLennan & Petty Pty Limited

Distributed in the United Kingdom
and Europe by
Blackwell Scientific Publications
Osney Mead, Oxford OX2 0EL
Orders should be addressed to:
Marston Book Services Ltd
PO Box 87
Oxford OX2 0DT
Tel: 0865 791155
Fax: 0865 791927
Telex: 837515

National Library of Australia
Cataloguing-in-Publication data:

Talley, Nicholas Joseph.
Examination medicine.
2nd ed.
Includes index.
ISBN 0 86433 068 5

1. Physical diagnosis
2. Physical diagnosis — Examinations, questions, etc.
I. O'Connor, Simon.    II. Title.
616.0754

Printed and bound in Australia

# Foreword

One hurdle that confronts all medical graduates who wish to specialize in medicine and its subspecialities is the examination for Fellowship of one of the Royal Colleges of Physicians. The anxiety and distortion of lifestyle that this examination provokes may create situations that interfere with the postgraduate training of medical graduates and overall render the examination counterproductive.

The aim of the book by Nicholas Talley and Simon O'Connor is to familiarize candidates with the examination, special emphasis being placed on medical problems that may be met. It is packed full of good advice and factual knowledge, and to read the book is an enjoyable as well as an instructive exercise.

To avoid errors that arise in single (or double) author books, the writers have had each branch of specialized knowledge reviewed by specialists in the field.

The book has the advantage that it fills a real need; also the data are correct and it is easily read. The writers are to be congratulated in their effort.

**D. W. Piper**

*Professor of Medicine*
*University of Sydney*

# Preface to the First Edition

*The life so short, the craft so long to learn*

Hippocrates (5th Century BC)

This book is written to help candidates sitting for the Royal Australasian College of Physicians (Part One) Examination. Much of the material has general application to physician training, particularly in the development of clinical skills. It is the masterly application of clinical skills, as well as the breadth of theoretical knowledge, that makes a doctor a consultant physician whose advice is sought by his or her colleagues.

We hope this book will help candidates understand what it means to be a physician. It is not intended to replace traditional textbooks, but rather to supplement them. Senior medical students who are interested in internal medicine will also find this book of value for their clinical examinations, but much theoretical knowledge is assumed. Paediatrics is not covered. Areas which candidates find most difficult (for example, neurological short cases) are discussed in greater detail in the text.

We sincerely hope our contribution will minimize the pain of preparing for the FRACP (Part One) examination.

# Preface to the Second Edition

Medicine is ever changing; indeed, many of the facts that we diligently committed to memory are no longer considered to be correct, and new pieces of information are continually being added. Still, the basic clinical skills of history taking and physical examination remain the cornerstone of current medical practice, and these skills must be mastered to obtain specialist qualifications. We have, therefore, been gratified by the success of the first edition of *Examination Medicine*; it has gained wide acceptance by candidates for the FRACP (Part One) for whom it is intended and has been well received by senior medical students.

In this edition we have completely revised and updated the text. New long cases have been added, and new lists of important facts have been incorporated. While this book emphasizes the clinical approach and describes how to elicit many important physical signs, the basics are not covered; we would suggest that readers refer to our book *Clinical Examination: A Guide to Physical Diagnosis* for further information. We have intentionally included humorous anecdotes, stories and cartoons, usually to illustrate an important point; while we cannot vouch for the exact authenticity of some of these, we firmly believe that studying medicine is optimized if it is also fun.

We wish you luck with your examination preparation.

**Nicholas Talley**
**Simon O'Connor**
*January 1991*

# Acknowledgements

The following specialists have been kind enough to review the appropriate sections of the second edition. We are very grateful for their advice and comments.

## CARDIOLOGY

**Dr M. Bell**, FRACP
Research Associate in Cardiology, Mayo Clinic, Rochester, Minnesota, USA.

**Dr D. L. Hayes**, MD
Associate Professor of Medicine and Consultant in Cardiology, Mayo Clinic, Rochester, Minnesota, USA.

## RESPIRATORY

**Dr M. Schonell**, FRACP, FRCP, FCCP
Visiting Respiratory Physician, St George Hospital, Sydney, Australia.

**Dr R. J. Pisani**, MD
Senior Associate Consultant in Thoracic Diseases, Mayo Clinic, Rochester, Minnesota, USA.

## GASTROENTEROLOGY

**Dr N. A. Talley**, FRACP
Director of Medicine and Visiting Gastroenterologist, St George Hospital, Sydney, Australia.

**Dr M. Camilleri**, MD, FRCP
Associate Professor of Medicine and Consultant in Gastroenterology, Mayo Clinic, Rochester, Minnesota, USA.

**Dr J. E. Clain**, MD
Associate Professor of Medicine and Consultant in Gastroenterology, Mayo Clinic, Rochester, Minnesota, USA.

## HAEMATOLOGY

**Dr A. Manoharan**, FRACP, FRCPA
Staff Specialist in Haematology, St George Hospital, Sydney, Australia.

**Dr D. A. Gastineau**, MD
Consultant in Haematology, Mayo Clinic, Rochester, Minnesota, USA.

## NEUROLOGY

**Dr P. G. McManis**, FRACP
Consultant in Neurology, Mayo Clinic, Rochester, Minnesota, USA.

**Dr G. Herkes**, FRACP
Fellow in Neurology, Mayo Clinic, Rochester, Minnesota, USA.

## RENAL DISEASE

**Dr M. Brown**, MD, FRACP
Staff Specialist in Renal Medicine and Senior Lecturer in Medicine, St George Hospital, Sydney, Australia.

**Dr T. R. Schwab**, MD
Consultant in Renal Medicine, Mayo Clinic, Rochester, Minnesota, USA.

## ENDOCRINOLOGY

**Dr T. T. Nguyen**, MD
Consultant in Endocrinology, Mayo Clinic, Rochester, Minnesota, USA.

**Dr P. Ebeling**, FRACP
Fellow in Endocrinology, Mayo Clinic, Rochester, Minnesota, USA.

## RHEUMATOLOGY

**Dr J. Edmonds**, FRACP
Professor of Rheumatology, St George Hospital, Sydney, Australia.

**Dr W. W. Ginsburg**, MD
Associate Professor of Medicine and Consultant in Rheumatology, Mayo Clinic, Rochester, Minnesota, USA.

## INFECTIOUS DISEASE

**Dr J. M. Steckelberg**, MD, FACP
Consultant in Infectious Disease, Mayo Clinic, Rochester, Minnesota, USA.

Despite all our best efforts, factual errors may still have been included. As with every book or authority, please check and question everything. Write to us if you have any suggestions.

# An Historical Note

*The problem is not so much how to test candidates
but how to test examinations.*

J. Parkhouse, *Lancet* 1971;i:905–6

Internal medicine at the beginning of this century was still in its infancy. It was practised largely on an empirical basis. Therapeutics was very limited. Surgery was a more popular speciality, partly because of its greater efficacy in treating many diseases. There were consultant physicians in Australia, but medicine was mainly practised by the family doctor.

In 1930 some leading physicians formed the Association of Physicians of Australia. It aimed to foster expansion of scientific knowledge of medicine in Australia and New Zealand. It also allowed physicians to meet socially. It was an exclusive organization—only physicians who held honorary appointments at teaching hospitals were eligible to join.

Non-members began to lobby, however, for the formation of a college. Eventually, after considerable opposition from members of the Association, the Royal Australasian College of Physicians was legally incorporated in 1938 (the title 'Royal' was conferred by King George VI). The inauguration ceremony occurred, with great pageantry, in the Great Hall of the University of Sydney. Sydney was chosen for the headquarters because the Royal Australasian College of Surgeons had previously been established in Melbourne.

Since the beginning, the College has been responsible for the maintenance of the standards of training and practice of medicine and paediatrics. This was originally achieved by conducting an examination known as 'the Membership'. The College set two major prerequisites for this test:

1. The candidate had to be a graduate of three or more years' standing from an acceptable medical school.
2. Two Fellows of the College vouched for the candidate's integrity and character.

No limits were set on age or experience, no attention was given to previous training, no standard was defined for the examination, and few guidelines were laid down. The Membership examination consisted of two papers of essay questions and a clinical and oral examination. Although this was a rather subjective test, Censors carried out their obligations well, as is obvious from the high standards of internal medicine practised in Australia and New Zealand today. Multiple-choice questions were introduced only in 1967.

With the growth of technology and medical knowledge, the College began to coordinate the flourishing speciality associations and societies. By 1968 the need for a change in evaluation of physician trainees became apparent. In 1976 the Membership examination was replaced by the Fellowship. After considerable discussion within the College, it was decided that the emphasis should be on training, rather than examination. To this end the FRACP (Part One) Examination was established as an early examination to admit candidates to advanced training. Candidates successful in this Part One Examination would then have three or four years of supervised training in general medicine or a subspeciality, and in most cases, no further examination would be required. An advanced trainee would be elected a Fellow after his or her required time of supervised training in accredited terms, if the supervisors' reports were satisfactory.

In this the College decided on a different course from the Royal Australasian College of Surgeons, which requires candidates to sit for an examination at the end of advanced training before election to Fellowship. The actual training emphasis of the Colleges still remains different.

Internal medicine today is an extremely popular speciality. The College of Physicians has helped promote ethical and professional standards, as well as the study of medicine. Influence has been extended to South-East Asia. Since 1963 teams have lectured in advanced medicine to postgraduates in Singapore with the University of Singapore. In 1966 the Asian-Pacific Committee was set up to ensure active participation in the maintenance of standards of medical education in the region. In

1976 the South-East Asian Regional Committee was set up to be responsible for meetings of College members in the region. As well, teachers have been sent to Kuala Lumpur (since 1975), and lecturers have been provided for the University of Papua New Guinea (since 1980).

Indeed, the FRACP (Part One) examination, with which this book deals, is now held at centres in Australia, New Zealand and Singapore.

The examination system has its critics. The pass rate for the FRACP (Part One) is low; in 1989 only 74 candidates (28%) passed both the written and their first attempt at the clinical examination. In the United Kingdom, the MRCP (UK) also has a low pass rate. In an editorial in *Lancet*, it was suggested there are only two possible reasons for a low pass rate in the MRCP: either the training or the examination is of poor quality and the College is directly or indirectly responsible for each (*Lancet* 1990; i:443–445). The Royal Australasian College of Physicians has tried to address some of these concerns in recent years. It now issues more comprehensive explanations of the aims and methods of its examinations, and unsuccessful candidates are sent a detailed explanation of their deficiencies.

The objectives of the College remain the same as they were at its inception. Essentially the College strives to promote the study of the art and science of medicine, encourage research and dissemination of knowledge, as well as *promote and ensure the fitness of persons desirous of qualifying for membership of the College*. This book deals with strategies to enable one to satisfy the strict examination requirements of the College.

# Contents

# Chapter 1

# BASIC TRAINING REQUIREMENTS

*I would live to study, and not study to live.*

Francis Bacon (1561–1626)

The requirements for basic training, after which the candidate may sit the Fellowship Examination, are set out in The Royal Australasian College of Physicians handbook, *Requirements for Physician Training*. These rules were changed in 1986 and are currently being reviewed again.

The College now requires three years of basic training after the intern year in Australia. In New Zealand training can begin after graduation, but the examination cannot be attempted until the third year of basic training at the earliest.

The College insists on at least 24 months of supervised training in general medicine or medical specialities ('core' training), which must involve the continuing care of medical patients in approved hospitals. Up to six months of this time may be undertaken in coronary care or other intensive units or both. Only six months may be spent in any one speciality. Part-time training, which has been approved by the College, is acceptable for a maximum of two years; details are available from the College.

Accreditation of terms as suitable for basic training has recently been made more difficult, and some hospitals have lost accreditation. This applies especially to hospitals which receive resident medical officers on secondment. Up to three months of core training may be carried out in an approved secondment post. It is important to check with the College Accreditation Committee if there is any doubt that terms are acceptable. It is wise to have this approval in writing. Basic training requirements are now so strict that careful negotiation with the hospital for suitable training terms from the beginning of basic training is the only way to ensure that it is possible to sit the examination in the minimum time.

A programme director (the coordinator of physician training) is appointed in each hospital which has an accredited training scheme. He or she is responsible for supervising basic training, and application forms for the examination are sent to him or her by the College.

Applications for the FRACP examination close at the end of November. It is not necessary to register for basic training with the College. All candidates are notified by post when their applications are received and again when approval to sit is granted. This second letter gives the times, date and place of the examination. In some cases, exemption from the written examination may be granted. This usually applies to people with postgraduate physician training and overseas qualifications—for example, the MRCP, the Diploma of the American Board of Internal Medicine, the FRCP (Canada), and the Master of Medicine (Singapore). The appropriate application form for exemption can be obtained from the College. Approval is not automatic but at the discretion of the Chief Censor. Exemption from the clinical examination will very occasionally be given to highly qualified senior people who trained overseas, but an interview is almost always required.

Candidates who have a higher degree (MD or PhD) may apply to have accred-ited one year of basic training or one year of advanced training.

The Part One FRACP examination is not recognized as a specialist qualification. To be admitted to Fellowship of the College requires completion of basic and advanced training and a pass in the Part One examination. Under the new rules, entry to advanced training no longer requires a pass in the examination. While specialist units prefer to appoint trainees who have passed the Part One, the option is available to appoint trainees who have completed basic training but not passed. Although candidates must eventually pass the examination, failure at the first attempt will not necessarily result in additional years of training. All advanced training in general medicine or a subspeciality must be approved by the appropriate Specialist Advisory Committee and by the Committee for Physician Training. At the end of each year, supervisors' reports are carefully reviewed, and a decision is made whether to accredit fully or partially, or not accredit, the advanced training. There is no longer any Part Two examination, but the College reserves the right to conduct one, or to insist on further training, if a candidate has performed inadequately during advanced training. This is a rare event. Advanced training requirements are very different for the various subspecialities, and details can be obtained from the College.

Determination to pass both sections of the examination at the first attempt is an important part of preparation. The first section is a written examination which is held only once every year, in February, in each of the Australian capital cities and in four main centres in New Zealand. The second part is a clinical *viva-voce* (live-voice) test. The clinical examinations can be attempted only by candidates who have been successful in the written part. Failure in the written examination means waiting a year to sit again. There is now no limit on the number of times one may sit the entire examination. Some persistent souls have sat many times (the record, we believe, is 11—and the candidate passed). Over 75% of these persons do eventually get through, if they have the stamina.

A list of successful candidates is published in the national press about one week after the examination, and the results are sent by facsimile to one location in each Australian and New Zealand centre on the day the results are determined. All candidates are notified by post also. Very occasionally a name can be left out of the paper—on one occasion an entire line of names was left out, but all the candidates concerned were notified by telegram and letter. Those who have failed the written examination are sent a computer-generated feedback sheet indicating their percentile ranking in the various speciality areas and in each section of the written paper. The coordinator of physician training of each hospital is sent a list of the average mark for the candidates from that hospital in each subspeciality.

The 'viva' examination is held twice each year—the first time in April and again in September of the same year as a 'post'. These 'vivas' are held in each capital city in rotation (for example, Sydney in September, Brisbane in April). This rotation forms the basis for the unofficial 'FRACP See Australia Travel Plan'. Experienced candidates know this tour well. In Australia, examinations are now held in both a major (Sydney, Melbourne, Brisbane or Adelaide) and a minor centre (Hobart, Canberra, Newcastle or Perth). The clinical exam is also available in Singapore. In Singapore candidates must have obtained the MMed (Singapore) in 1987 or later. The test there involves teams of examiners, including at least one representative of the Committee for Examinations from Australia and New Zealand, and the examination is held after the clinical MMed Singapore exams, which are in June. In 1989 for the first time in living memory the 'viva' was postponed in Australia for two months because of a pilots' strike. Such events cannot be relied upon to give more time for preparation. A pass in April or September counts as a pass in the year the written examination was sat.

The cost of travel and accommodation must be added to the examination fee. The current fee is $A800, which is for the written examination and the April 'viva'. Failure in April entitles the candidate to sit again in September, but the fee is charged again. The claiming of these expenses as a tax concession is being reviewed by the Taxation Commission, but usually seems to be allowed.

An exemption from the written examination usually entitles the candidate to sit the 'viva' in September only, not in April. Failure in September means sitting the written examination again.

The practice of putting up results in one location on the same day has now been reintroduced. The story goes that the practice was abandoned in the 1970s because a few candidates tied knots in the chains of the Grandfather clock and did other damage necessitating the repainting of the lobby of the Royal College of Surgeons where the results were to be posted! Currently results will be posted at 6 o'clock at a location which will be advised; it is usually at the site of the examiners' meeting. A list of successful candidates from the 'viva' examination is also published in the national press within a week. Notification by post comes a little later.

Unsuccessful candidates receive a list describing the deficiencies found (for example, 'unsatisfactory examination of the cardiovascular system'). This indicates which cases the candidate has failed. The College also sends a detailed critique of the candidate's performance from the notes which are made by the four examiners during the 10-minute period provided for discussion of a candidate's performance.

Successful candidates receive a letter of congratulations, and an application form to join the College as an advanced trainee. The *Handbook of Physician Training* is also sent.

For further information write to one of the following:

Honorary Secretary
The Royal Australasian College of Physicians
145 Macquarie Street
Sydney, NSW 2000
AUSTRALIA

Honorary Secretary
New Zealand Committee
The Royal Australasian College of Physicians
Kevin Chambers, 16 The Terrace
Wellington 1
NEW ZEALAND

# Chapter 2
# THE WRITTEN EXAMINATION

*No man's opinions are better than his information.*

Paul Getty (1960)

## THE EXAMINATION FORMAT

The written examination is a screening examination to select candidates for further testing. Like Caesar's Gaul, it is divided into three parts. These are all held on the same day. It is an objective multiple-choice examination. There are five choices in each question, any of which can be true or false, and there is always at least one correct answer. Each part is designed to test a separate fact, so they are often quite distinct from each other. Marks are deducted for all wrong answers. In any question, if three or more parts are answered incorrectly, a negative mark will be given for the entire question. A pencil is provided at the test, as well as a well-used eraser. It is advisable, however, to bring a pencil sharpener, a spare soft B pencil, and a good eraser.

The marking system is complex. All questions are approved by a test committee. There is unfortunately no predetermined pass mark. All candidates' papers are first scored. Any question which most people mark correctly may be eliminated as too easy. Any question which most candidates get wrong may also be eliminated as too difficult. The best questions discriminate between the 'good' and 'bad' candidates. Then various statistical methods are employed to separate candidates into two groups. The exact pass mark is set at approximately one-quarter standard deviation below the mean mark for Australasia, in such a way that the cut-off falls in a gap between clusters of candidates. Approximately 60% to 70% are in the 'good' group, and these people pass. This means one must aim to be better than at least 40% of the other candidates to be successful. The pass mark is not set according to the number of places available in the clinicals.

The examination is no longer held in winter, but experienced candidates could be spotted in the past at the Sydney centre because they came equipped with coats, scarves and thick woollen socks. (For some reason the examination room at the

University of Sydney was not heated.) This problem has been solved by changing the date of the examination.

Paper A (which is given first, usually at 9:00 a.m.) tests the principles of medicine. There are also some questions which test the application of the basic sciences (particularly physiology) to clinical medicine. Two hours are allowed. There are 60 questions. A more physiological flavour to the test has been apparent in recent years.

A short break follows the first paper; then, somewhat surprisingly, comes Paper C. There is always one electrocardiogram and often one echocardiogram; hypertrophic cardiomyopathy is always popular. Various X-ray films (including chest radiographs), blood films (actual photographs or reports or both), photographs of urinary sediment and histopathology slides (for example, a renal biopsy slide) are usually included. Photographs (in both black and white and colour) are usually of high quality. Interpretation of biochemistry results (for example, liver function tests) is also examined. Normal values are always supplied. This ordeal lasts one and a half hours and there are 33 questions.

A break of one hour for lunch (for those with an appetite) is followed by Paper B in the afternoon. This examines the practice of medicine and therapeutics and has 60 questions. The time allowed is two and a half hours.

# APPROACHING MULTIPLE-CHOICE QUESTIONS

By the time they sit this examination, most candidates will have had considerable experience with multiple-choice questions. However, it is worth stating a few relevant points.

There is very rarely any shortage of time, and therefore, there is no need to hurry. The questions are complicated and each tests several pieces of knowledge. The correct answer may be a number of steps removed from the initial statement. All this is an indication of the importance of reading each question with great care and looking especially for negatives and double negatives. Most people find their first carefully considered answer is more reliable than a change of mind on later review of the paper.

It is worth remembering that the words 'always' and 'never' do not often apply in medicine. The word 'recognized' means that an association has been described, whereas 'characteristic' implies that the given factor is important to the condition and essential to the diagnosis.

It is probably better to guess at answers where the question is obscure than to leave a question out entirely. To avoid coming to the end of the paper and finding an unfilled space on the answer sheet, a constant check that question and answer numbers match is desirable.

# PREPARATION FOR
# THE WRITTEN EXAMINATION

The College does not send a curriculum for the written examination, but recommends the use of any major textbook and some journals (see Further Reading). The authors have found that concentrating on the latest edition of a standard textbook (for example, the most recent edition of Harrison's *Principles of Internal Medicine* or the *Oxford Textbook of Medicine*) to be a most satisfactory method of preparation. The *Medical Knowledge Self Assessment Program* (*MKSAP*) of the American College of Physicians is also available. It contains brief up-to-date accounts of most areas of internal medicine. It clearly indicates the currently fashionable topics on which questions are likely to be set. It also has a comprehensive series of multiple-choice questions based on the text. Only some of these questions are of a similar standard to the Part One written examination questions.

The College now produces its own self-assessment questions—the *Australian Self Assessment Programme* (*ASAP*). These *ASAP* questions are produced every three years and can be highly recommended. None of the questions is likely to appear in the examination paper, as the *ASAP* is primarily educational and, therefore, tends to have a bias towards positive responses, unlike the Part One examination.

There is great value in practising multiple-choice questions. Sample questions from papers A, B, and C are available from the College. These are taken from papers used in recent years and represent questions considered to have discriminating value. The Committee for Examinations also releases, every second year, complete copies of written examination papers set three years previously. Old questions do not usually appear in the examination paper. The College has a large bank of questions which are adjusted annually. The Written Examination Committee adds new questions and updates and improves old questions.

Many hospitals conduct their own trial examination with questions written by the staff. There are also books of multiple-choice questions available on the market, which are based on other postgraduate examinations like the MRCP, but they are of much less value.

Practising multiple-choice questions with a group of three or four to discuss the various options is found helpful by many candidates.

The College recommends a number of general medicine journals that candidates should read regularly (p. 258). The authors recommend concentrating on editorials and review articles. Study of specialist journals is not required.

Postgraduate institutions hold courses on various topics before the examinations which some candidates may find helpful. A course of lectures lasting 34 weeks (one night per week for 17 weeks per year over 2 years) is available for the Part One candidates in Sydney. Such courses are also available in New Zealand.

There are a number of cassette tape programmes available on medical topics, including the Royal Australasian College of Physicians *Recent Advances in Medicine*, available from the Continuing Education Centre. Current topics include mitral

valve prolapse, antiarrhythmic drugs, hypertension, the many faces of lupus, pituitary tumours, a pragmatic approach to anaemia, and difficult pneumonias. These
are available from the College.

In summary, we have listed a number of conventional but important suggestions
for the written examination:

1. Be well rested and avoid travelling long distances on the eve of the examination.
2. Be familiar with the format of the paper and know how much time to allow
   for each question.
3. Work through the paper at a leisurely, deliberate pace and return to troub-
   lesome questions at the end. Inspiration may well come from other questions.
4. Rely on first careful impressions and do not change an answer if there is
   doubt.
5. Check every tenth question or so to be sure that answers match the question
   numbers.
6. Have a short rest after the written examination, but begin work for the 'viva'
   examination before the results come out, as time is very limited between the
   two parts of the examination.

# Chapter 3

# SUGGESTED TOPICS FOR
# THE WRITTEN EXAMINATION

*Every physician, almost, hath his favourite disease.*

*Tom Jones*, Henry Fielding (1707–1754)

## INTRODUCTION

The authors have compiled, in this section, an INCOMPLETE list of topics from their own and colleagues' experience of the written examination over the last several years. However, greater breadth and depth of knowledge are required to pass. Many have found such a list a very useful method of checking progress, and it may also help those who would not otherwise have realized that certain areas (for example, psychiatry or basic physiology) are examined in the Part One written test.

The closing date for multiple-choice question submissions is approximately four months before the examination sitting date. After detailed evaluation, the actual questions are selected in December or January. Remember that any fashionable topic (for example, Lyme arthritis or acquired immune deficiency syndrome—AIDS) which has appeared in the popular press in the year prior to the closing date may crop up.

We strongly believe that seeing many cases for the clinical part is a very good way of reinforcing theoretical knowledge. Many physicians base their knowledge on cases seen personally.

Do not concentrate on strong areas or only on topics of great interest. This is a certain way to be unsuccessful. Questions are drawn from all branches of medicine, especially the large subspecialities. Medicine relevant to the South-East Asian region is also sometimes examined.

Some areas appear only very rarely in the test (for example, statistics, genetics, or unusual tropical diseases).

# IMPORTANT TOPICS

## Papers A and B

We have combined the topics from papers A and B, as they are very similar and complementary.

### *Cardiovascular System* (pp. 33–51, 135–160)

*Physical Examination*

e.g., pulse character, jugular venous pressure waves, abnormal heart sounds, clinical signs of severity of valve lesions.

*Anatomy*

e.g., coronary arteries.

*Physiology*

e.g., metabolic substrate for heart muscle, red blood cells, and skeletal muscle.

*Non-invasive Tests*

e.g., exercise stress test interpretation, Bayes' theorum, ECG changes in different conditions such as pericarditis or right ventricular infarction.

*Chronic Coronary Heart Disease*

e.g., coronary artery spasm, causes of non-atherosclerotic angina, ischaemic cardio-myopathy, coronary artery bypass grafting, left internal mammary artery grafting, coronary angioplasty.

*Acute Myocardial Infarction*

e.g., measurement of infarct size, right ventricular infarction (features and prognosis), thrombolysis (agents, indications and contraindications), anaesthetic risks following infarction, early complications of infarction, assessment of risk.

*Arrhythmias*

e.g., supraventricular tachycardia and its mechanisms, ventricular tachycardia and its mechanisms, antiarrhythmic drugs, electrical approaches for treatment of lethal ventricular arrhythmias using automatic, implantable cardioverter-defibrillators.

*Valvular Heart Disease*

e.g., mitral valve prolapse, prosthetic heart valves, valvular heart disease and pregnancy.

*Infective Endocarditis*

e.g., organisms, diagnostic features, complications.

*Cardiomyopathy*
e.g., hypertrophic cardiomyopathy.

*Pericardial Disease*
e.g., viral causes, Dressler's syndrome (features and complications).

*Congenital Heart Disease*
e.g., atrial septal defect, ventricular septal defect, patent ductus arteriosus, Ebstein's anomaly, Fallot's tetralogy, Eisenmenger's syndrome, bicuspid aortic valve, coarctation of the aorta.

*Pulmonary Heart Disease*
e.g., pulmonary hypertension, pulmonary embolism.

*Peripheral Vascular Disease*
e.g., acute aortic dissection and its associations.

*Hypertension*
e.g., complications.

*Congestive Cardiac Failure*
e.g., ejection fraction, mechanisms of oedema, benefits of drug treatment, cardiac transplant, physiology of pulmonary oedema.

*Cardiac Catheterization*
e.g., pressures and saturations—interpretation.

*Shock*
e.g., the major endogenous mediator in sepsis (cachectin or tumour necrosis factor), multi-organ failure, prognosis.

## Respiratory System (pp. 51–64, 160–176)

*Lung Mechanics*
e.g., pleural pressures, elastic recoil, cough syncope.

*Physiology*
e.g., haemoglobin affinity for oxygen.

*Chronic Obstructive Pulmonary Disease*
e.g., elastic properties of the lung in emphysema, poor prognostic features, causes of hypoventilation, effect on the pulmonary circulation.

*Asthma*
e.g., bronchopulmonary aspergillosis and its importance, precipitating factors, desensitization treatment, RAST testing, late-phase reactions.

*Small Airways Disease*

*Sleep Disorders*
e.g., obstructive sleep apnoea, central apnoea.

*Interstitial Lung Disease*
e.g., silicosis (diagnosis and features), sarcoidosis, pulmonary fibrosis, drug causes, bronchoalveolar lavage.

*Infectious Disease*
e.g., pneumococcal vaccine, non-bacterial pneumonia, Legionella, fungal disease, tuberculosis, human immunodeficiency virus (HIV) and the lung.

*Occupational Lung Disease*
e.g., asbestosis (including relationship to the amount of exposure and the different types).

*Genetic Defects*
e.g., cystic fibrosis (diagnosis, management and prognosis), immotile cilia syndrome.

*Lung Neoplasms*
e.g., smoking association, additive risk factors, different cell types and their different presentations, mesothelioma.

*Pulmonary Embolus*
e.g., features, diagnosis and effects.

*Rhinitis*
e.g., causes, control.

*Vasculitis*
e.g., Wegener's granulomatosis treatment.

*Adult Respiratory Distress Syndrome*

*Pneumothorax*
e.g., spontaneous pneumothorax, incidence, recurrence, associations and treatment.

*Pleural Disease*
e.g., mesothelioma.

*Lung Transplantation*

## Gastrointestinal System (pp. 64–80, 165, 177–182)

*Oesophagus*
e.g., achalasia, diffuse oesophageal spasm, reflux, drugs which change lower oesophageal sphincter pressures, Barrett's oesophagus, motor activity.

## Stomach

e.g., *Helicobacter pylori* gastritis, side effects of $H_2$-receptor blockers and omeprazole, gastrointestinal hormones (especially gastrin, cholecystokinin and secretin), control of acid secretion, gastric carcinoma, haemorrhage and the role of endoscopy.

## Small Intestine

e.g., fat absorption mechanisms, diagnostic uses of small bowel biopsy, bacterial overgrowth syndromes, vitamin $B_{12}$ malabsorption, intestinal lactase deficiency, coeliac disease.

## Large Intestine

e.g., antibiotic-associated colitis, inflammatory bowel disease, solitary ulcer in the colon, reactive arthritis.

## Pancreas

e.g., hyperamylasaemia, chronic pancreatitis.

## Liver and Biliary Tract

e.g., causes of chronic liver disease, associations of chronic active hepatitis, haemochromatosis, Wilson's disease, hepatitis (B and C), causes of hepatic granulomas, alpha-1 antitrypsin deficiency (genetics and effects), bile secretion (e.g., conjugation, phospholipid content), liver transplantation, physiology of ascites, cholangitis, hepatitis B vaccine.

## Diarrhoea

e.g., *Yersinia* enterocolitis, traveller's diarrhoea, *Clostridium difficile*, gay bowel syndrome.

## Trace Elements

e.g., zinc deficiency

# Haematology (pp. 80–92, 182–185)

## Red Cell Indices

e.g., causes of change in mean corpuscular volume (MCV).

## Anaemia

e.g., types, causes, Coomb's test interpretation.

## Haemopoietic Stem Cell Disorders

e.g., preleukaemic syndromes, myeloproliferative diseases (polycythaemia rubra vera—distinguishing primary and secondary types, chronic myeloid leukaemia, essential thrombocythaemia, myelofibrosis).

*Erythropoiesis and Disorders of Red Cells*
e.g., causes of hypochromic anaemia, iron metabolism, aplastic anaemia, haemolytic anaemia, causes of iron deficiency, vitamin $B_{12}$ and folate metabolism, thalassaemia (complications, types), hereditary spherocytosis.

*Granulopoiesis and Disorders of White Cells*
e.g., causes of eosinophilia, eosinophil function, eosinophilia-myalgia syndrome.

*Multiple Myeloma*
e.g., diagnosis, complications.

*Lymphopoiesis and Disorders of Lymphocytes*
e.g., angioimmunoblastic lymphadenopathy, lymphoma (types and treatment), myeloma and dysproteinaemias, acute lymphoblastic leukaemia—cytological features and prognosis.

*Haemostasis Defects*
e.g., platelets—congenital defects (Bernard-Soulier's disease, Glanzmann's disease, von Willebrand's disease), haemophilia, lupus anticoagulant, protein C and S deficiency, antithrombin III deficiency, interpretation of coagulation tests, heparin-induced thrombocytopenia.

*Splenectomy*
e.g., indications and complications.

*Bone Marrow Transplantation*

## Nervous System (pp. 122–128, 205–251)

*Electrodiagnosis*
e.g., electromyography (EMG)—fibrillation potentials and disease findings, electroencephalograms (EEG), caloric responses, brain death diagnosis.

*Cerebrospinal Fluid*
e.g., immunoglobulin changes with disease.

*Anatomy*
e.g., spinal cord pain pathways, diagnostic possibilities regarding brain biopsy (pathology)

*Dementia*
e.g., reversible causes.

*Encephalopathy*

*Vision*
e.g., causes of unilateral visual loss, causes of bilateral visual loss, visual evoked responses.

*Muscle Disease*
e.g., myasthenia gravis, dystrophia myotonica, electromyography (EMG) interpretation.

*Cerebrovascular Disease*
e.g., cerebral haemorrhages—common sites and causes, features of internal carotid artery occlusion, transient ischaemic attack features and causes, aphasia, transient global amnesia, lacunar infarcts.

*Organic Brain Syndromes*
e.g., neurological features of liver failure.

*Headache*
e.g., cluster headache, migraine.

*Nystagmus*
e.g., causes and types.

*Tumours*
e.g., cerebellopontine angle tumour (and caloric findings).

*Extrapyramidal Syndromes*
e.g., chorea.

*Peripheral Nerve Injuries*

*Drugs*
e.g., neurological findings with drug overdose, anti-Parkinsonian drugs.

*Cerebral Abscess*
e.g., causes and features.

## Psychiatry

*Schizophrenia*
e.g., inheritance, risk to relatives, possible causes of schizophrenic-like illnesses.

*Organic Psychoses*
e.g., distinguishing hypomania from organic psychoses by clinical features and EEG.

*Depression*
e.g., difference from dementia.

*Panic Attacks*
e.g., recognition, treatment, risk of benzodiazepines.

*Anorexia Nervosa and Bulimia*
e.g., diagnosis.

*Defence Mechanisms*
e.g., sublimation.

*Drugs—Mechanism of Action and Side Effects*
e.g., major tranquilizers, antidepressants (tricyclic, tetracyclic and MAO inhibitors), lithium.

## Rheumatology (pp. 92–105, 200–205)

*Biology of Connective Tissue*
e.g., different types of collagen.

*Rheumatoid Arthritis*
e.g., serology (nature of rheumatoid factor, antinuclear factor), X-ray findings, complications, other causes of polyarthritis, juvenile rheumatoid arthritis (types, clinical features), drugs (particularly methotrexate, gold, penicillamine, chloroquine).

*Raynaud's Phenomenon*
e.g., associations.

*Sjögren's Syndrome*
e.g., SS-A and SS-B antibody associations, association with lymphoma.

*Systemic Lupus Erythematosus*
e.g., nervous system complications, problems with pregnancy, anti-cardiolipin antibodies, features of drug-induced lupus.

*Systemic Sclerosis*
e.g., differential diagnosis.

*Seronegative Arthropathy*
e.g., Behçet's syndrome features, diagnosis of Reiter's syndrome, HLA-B27 association with each disease, intestinal bypass surgery—associations, Whipple's disease.

*Osteoarthritis*
e.g., primary osteoarthritis—synovial fluid characteristics, pathogenesis and X-ray changes.

*Haemochromatosis Arthropathy*

*Vasculitis*
e.g., giant cell arteritis and association with polymyalgia rheumatica, Wegener's granulomatosis, mixed cryoglobulinaemia, Henöch-Schönlein purpura.

*Crystal-Induced Synovitis*
e.g., crystal characteristics of gout, pseudogout and hydroxyapatite arthropathy.

*Infectious Arthritis*
e.g., Lyme arthritis, gonococcal arthritis.

*Non-steroidal Anti-Inflammatory Drugs*
e.g., prevention of gastric damage using misoprostol.

## *Infectious Diseases* (pp. 128–131)

*Fever*
e.g., mechanisms, types.

*Viral Diseases*
e.g., Epstein-Barr virus (association with Burkitt's lymphoma and nasopharyngeal carcinoma, complications including cranial nerve palsies, diagnosis), herpes simplex (complications including encephalitis, diagnosis, treatment), measles (complications, diagnosis), arboviruses (e.g., dengue fever), viral gastroenteritis (e.g., *E. coli* 0157:H7, rotavirus incubation period and diagnosis), enterovirus (acute haemorrhagic conjunctivitis), influenza, slow viruses (e.g., Jakob-Creutzfeldt disease, pathological findings, sterilization of instruments), teratogenic viruses, HIV infection (seroconversion and clinical disease, risks after needle stick, effects of azidothymidine).

*Bacterial Diseases*
e.g., gram-negative aerobes (e.g., *Campylobacter jejuni* clinical features and treatment), anaerobes (e.g., *Clostridium difficile* and its toxin, *Bacteroides fragilis*), mycobacterial infection (including atypical mycobacterium), Lyme disease, mycotic disease (e.g., cryptococcosis, aspergillosis), parasitic diseases (e.g., resistant strains of malaria, exoerythrogenic phases and types, transmission, treatment, drugs interfering with thick films), *Pneumocystis carinii* (organism, diagnosis, treatment).

*Syphilis Serology*

*Worms*
e.g., appearance of hookworms, roundworms; worms known to migrate; worms which cause eosinophilia.

*Antibiotics*
e.g., antibiotics which induce L forms of bacteria, importance of beta-lactamase production.

*Vaccines*
e.g., hepatitis B vaccine, dangers and value.

*Diseases in Specific Populations*
e.g., homosexual men—particularly AIDS and gay bowel syndrome, immunocompromised hosts.

*Other Topics*
e.g., organisms persisting after primary infections (as in varicella, tuberculosis), bacterial endotoxins and exotoxins, Kawasaki disease, non-specific urethritis, toxic shock syndrome, blood cultures——diagnostic valve in aerobic and anaerobic infections.

## Oncology

*Tumour Induction*
e.g., cigarettes, benzene, Epstein-Barr virus.

*Tumour-Associated Markers*
e.g., alpha-fetoprotein, carcinoembryonic antigen, prostate-specific antigen, beta human chorionic gonadotrophin (HCG).

*Antitumour Drugs*
e.g., mode of action and side effects of each.

*Breast Carcinoma*
e.g., oestrogen receptor status importance, role of adjuvant therapy, treatment of disseminated disease.

*Prostatic Carcinoma*
e.g., acid phosphatase test reliability.

*Colon Carcinoma*
e.g., adjuvant therapy, treatment for metastases.

*Malignant Melanoma*
e.g., poor prognostic features, new chemotherapeutic approaches.

*Retinoblastoma*
e.g., inheritance, prognosis.

*Radiotherapy*
e.g., indications, mechanisms of action, complications.

*Testicular Tumours*
e.g., common types, investigations, treatment.

*Sarcomas*
e.g., with Paget's disease, radiosensitivity.

*Manifestations of Cancer*
e.g., paraneoplastic syndromes, neurological manifestations, superior vena cava syndrome, malignant effusions, infection in the compromised host, common metastatic sites.

*Biological Response Modifiers*
e.g., interferons.

## *Endocrine* (pp. 105–113, 185–200)

*Hormonal Activity*
e.g., sites of action, receptor sites.

*Anterior Pituitary Lobe*
e.g., diagnostic tests of function, 'empty sella' syndrome, prolactin-secreting tumours.

*Posterior Pituitary Lobe*
e.g., antidiuretic hormone—structure, drugs affecting levels, psychogenic polydipsia.

*Ectopic Hormone Secretion*

*Adrenal Cortex*
e.g., Cushing's syndrome tests; aldosterone—stimulators and inhibitors of secretion, sites of production, synthesis; Addison's disease and its associations, risk of antibiotics inducing adrenal insufficiency.

*Adrenal Medulla*
e.g., phaeochromocytoma.

*Thyroid Gland*
e.g., T4, T3, reverse T3, sensitive TSH changes in health and disease, drugs affecting conversion of T4 to T3, multinodular goitre, de Quervain's thyroiditis, thyroxine replacement, management of hypothyroid states, eye disorders in Grave's disease, congenital hypothyroidism.

*Reproductive System*
e.g., causes of gynaecomastia, infertility and galactorrhoea, testosterone-binding activity and control of secretion, hormonal control of spermatogenesis, hirsutism, Klinefelter's syndrome.

*Bone and Mineral Disorders*
e.g., primary hyperparathyroidism, biochemical features in various diseases, vitamin D metabolism, oestrogen therapy in postmenopausal women (indications, risks).

*Atrial Natriuretic Factor*
e.g., effects, site of origin.

*Diabetes Mellitus*
e.g., biochemical control of gluconeogenesis, insulin antibodies, viruses associated with diabetes, reversible abnormalities in diabetes (e.g., red cell deformability, capillary leaks, triglycerides, neuropathy), drugs causing diabetes, pathogenesis of

ketoacidosis, hypoglycaemia and its association with immunoreactive insulin, gestational diabetes, glycosylated proteins, treatment of retinopathy, characteristics of amyotrophy, detecting incipient nephropathy.

*Anorexia Nervosa*
e.g., endocrine changes.

*Hormones and Growth*
e.g., effects on skeletal maturity, somatomedins (including IGF-1), growth hormone.

*Gynaecomastia*
e.g., hormonal and drug causes.

*HIV and Endocrinological Complications*

## Renal System (pp. 113–122, 179)

*Electrolyte and Water Disturbances*
e.g., inappropriate antidiuretic hormone secretion, diabetes insipidus, sodium disorders, potassium disorders, calcium disorders, countercurrent multiplication and exchange.

*Acid-Base Disturbances*
e.g., metabolic acidosis and alkalosis, causes of an increased, normal and low anion gap.

*Urinary Protein Excretion*
e.g., nephrotic syndrome.

*Urine Microscopy*

*Glomerulonephritis*
e.g., classification, IgA nephropathy, complement changes, Goodpasture's syndrome, nephritic and nephrotic syndromes.

*Systemic Diseases*
e.g., vasculitis, diabetes and systemic lupus erythematosus in the kidney.

*Tubulointestitial Nephritis*
e.g., causes, clinical course.

*Hypertension*
e.g., causes, plasma renin levels in various disorders, natriuretic hormones, therapy.

*Drugs and the Kidney*
e.g., safe antibiotics to prescribe in renal failure, effects of non-steroidal anti-inflammatory drugs in renal failure, analgesic nephropathy.

*Chronic Renal Failure*
e.g., reversible causes, manifestations, treatment (e.g., erythropoietin, transplantation, dialysis), polycystic disease.

*Acute Renal Failure*

*Renal Stones and Hypercalciuria*

*Urinary Tract Infection*
e.g., urinary incontinence, urinary catheterization.

*Bartter's Syndrome*

*Rhabdomyolysis*

*Pregnancy and the Kidney*

## Clinical Pharmacology

*Ionizaton of Drugs and Movement Across Membranes*
e.g., drugs with lipid solubility.

*Dose-Response Curve*
e.g., competitive and non-competitive antagonists.

*Drug Receptors*
e.g., alteration with chronic therapy.

*Cardiovascular System and Drugs*
e.g., alpha and beta effects of catecholamines, diuretics (site of action), digoxin (differences from digitoxin and ouabain, effects of intoxication), antihypertensive drugs (e.g., withdrawal hypertension), antiarrhythmic drugs (classes and effects, proarrhythmic effects, contraindications), cholesterol and drugs.

*Respiratory System and Drugs*
e.g., aminophylline ($t_{1/2}$ in different conditions).

*Gastrointestinal System and Drugs*
e.g., drugs that promote healing of peptic ulcer, paracetamol toxicity, side effects of laxatives.

*Haematological System and Drugs*
e.g., warfarin (how levels are increased or decreased and the causes of such changes), heparin (antibodies, toxicity), folate antagonists.

*Nervous System and Drugs*
e.g., L-dopa (contraindications, side effects), neurotoxic antibodies, cholinergic and anti-cholinergic drugs.

*Endocrine System and Drugs*

e.g., drugs precipitating diabetes mellitus (e.g., diuretics, diazoxide, phenytoin), prednisone (side effects, $t_{1/2}$ compared with other steroid agents), general effects of steroids, vitamin D (metabolism, effects on parathyroid hormone and calcium).

*Psychiatry and Drugs*

e.g., neuroleptic drugs (mechanisms of action, side effects), lithium (absorption, indications, routine management).

*Antibiotics*

e.g., penicillin G (mode of action, structure, effect of renal failure), sulphonylureas (side effects), metronidazole, cephalosporins, imipenem, fluoroquinolones.

*Antiviral Agents*

e.g., indications, treatment of HIV infection.

*Cytotoxic Drugs*

e.g., adriamycin (mechanism of action, usefulness, cardiotoxicity, monitoring), methotrexate (indications, interaction with salicylates, activation, protein binding, excretion, antagonistic factors, side effects including monitoring for liver toxicity), cyclophosphamide (absorption, mechanism of action), azathioprine (use in pregnancy, $t_{1/2}$), 5-fluorouracil (mode of action, administration, indications, complications), cell cycle-specific drugs.

*Other Topics*

e.g., heroin withdrawal features, drugs affecting free water clearance (e.g., increased by ethanol and lithium, decreased by nicotine, vincristine and clofibrate), pharmacology of alcohol and tobacco.

*Genetically Determined Drug Reactions*

e.g., malignant hyperpyrexia, succinylcholine apnoea.

*Pregnancy*

e.g., physiological changes, effect on chronic disease, drug use in, cholestasis.

# Paper C

## *Cardiovascular System* (pp. 135–59)

Electrocardiogram—usually only one, e.g., a combination of atrial fibrillation, right bundle branch block and left anterior hemiblock.
Chest X-ray films, e.g., left ventricular aneurysm.
2D and M-mode echocardiogram, e.g., hypertrophic cardiomyopathy, septal motion abnormalities, normal anatomy.
Coronary angiography (the different views and the names of the main vessels and their branches).

## Respiratory System (pp. 160–3)

Chest X-ray film, e.g., silicosis, bronchiectasis.
Respiratory function tests, e.g., $FEV_1$ (forced expiratory volume in 1 second), FVC (forced vital capacity), maximal voluntary ventilation, diffusing capacity.
Arterial blood gas level interpretation, e.g., significance of alveolar-arterial differences.
Ventilation-perfusion scan interpretation, e.g., pulmonary embolus.

## Gastrointestinal System

Barium swallow, e.g., achalasia, diffuse oesophageal spasm, stricture.
Barium meal, e.g., linitis plastica.
Barium enema, e.g., inflammatory bowel disease.
Abdominal CT scans, e.g., normal anatomy, lymphoma, pancreatic cancer.
Small intestinal biopsy findings, e.g., coeliac disease.
Malabsorption test interpretation, e.g., bacterial overgrowth.
Liver tests, e.g., assessment of a jaundiced patient, interpretation of hepatitis serology.

## Haematological System

Full blood count reports, e.g., features of acute lymphocytic leukaemia.
Blood film photographs, e.g., microcytic anaemia, liver disese.
Iron studies, e.g., interpret serum iron level, total iron-binding capacity, and serum ferritin level.
Protein electrophoresis, e.g., alpha-1 antitrypsin deficiency.
Coagulation tests.

## Central Nervous System

Carotid angiography and duplex scanning.
CT and MRI scans of the brain, e.g., normal anatomy.
Electromyograph (EMG) findings, e.g., distinguishing peripheral neuropathy from myopathy.
Electroencephalogram (EEG)—interpretation of reports.
Visual-evoked responses.

## Renal System

Intravenous pyelograms, e.g., polycystic kidney disease.
CT scans, e.g., polycystic kidney disease.
Bone radiographs, e.g., hips with renal osteodystrophy.
Urine sediment photograph, e.g., red and white cell casts.
Renal biopsy photographs, e.g., crescentic glomerulonephritis, vasculitis.

## Endocrine System

Pituitary function tests.
Thyroid function tests.
Diagnosis of Cushing's syndrome.
Electrolyte changes, e.g., Addison's disease.

### *Rheumatology*

Joint radiographs, e.g., hands in gouty arthropathy, fingers in psoriatic arthritis.
Synovial fluid analysis.

### *Immunology*

Complement findings in disease.

### *Infectious Diseases*

Cerebrospinal fluid findings, e.g., meningitis.
Syphilis serology interpretation.
Gallium and indium scans.

Chapter 4

# AN APPROACH TO
# THE CLINICAL EXAMINATION

*For one mistake made for not knowing,*
*ten mistakes are made for not looking.*

J. A. Lindsay

This is a very testing part. It is more difficult than the written test.

## THE EXAMINATION FORMAT

The clinical examination consists of two parts: (i) the long case; (ii) the short cases. Candidates are notified of the starting time of the ordeal, usually on green paper, after their success in the written papers. Be on time; the examination runs to a strict timetable and no time can be allowed for late arrival.

The long case is always first. At the appropriate moment candidates are escorted to the patient by a 'bulldog'. The word 'bulldog' is apparently derived from the name of Proctor's attendants at the universities of Oxford and Cambridge. He or she is usually a resident medical officer working at the examining hospital who has an interest in sitting the Part One examination. If ever candidates have the opportunity to work as a 'bulldog', then it should be taken. The 'bulldog' will introduce the candidate to the patient and then leave. There are never any examiners in the room during a long case. The time is limited to 65 minutes with the patient. A five-minute warning will be given after 60 minutes. At the end, candidates are escorted by the 'bulldog' from the patient's room to a chair outside the examiners' room. There, five further minutes are allowed for candidates to pull themselves together. A glass of water or weak orange juice is usually offered at this stage. If this does not occur, do ask for a drink if in need.

A bell will then ring and the candidate is taken in, seated, and introduced to the examiners. Try to appear self-possessed (even if weak at the knees), but don't give an air of nonchalance (e.g., don't slouch in your chair).

25

As a rule there are three examiners, but there may only be two. One is a member of the Court of Clinical Examiners. One or two others are experienced examiners who are local physicians, including perhaps the coordinator of Physician Training. There may be a small audience of 'bulldogs' as well. For reasons of fairness, it is unusual for specialists to examine a candidate in their own field. Twenty-two minutes are spent with the examiners, presenting the case and discussing diagnosis and management. They will assess the candidate's knowledge, attitude, personality, interpretive abilities, problem-solving abilities and clinical techniques. Only two examiners will ask questions—usually one 'leads' the discussion and the other follows near the end.

At the end of the time a bell will ring and the candidate is almost immediately taken to begin the short case examination. There are approximately two or three minutes, however, for weak orange juice. Many candidates ask the 'bulldog's' opinion of their performance. We believe this to be an unwise policy as the resident medical officer is usually junior to the examinee and so is often incorrect in his or her assessment.

The candidate is then introduced to the short case examiners. These examiners are never the same as the ones who examined for the long case. Again, one examiner is usually a College censor. A total of 22 minutes is allowed for the short cases. It is important to remember that there is no fixed number of cases that must be seen in this time to pass. Candidates usually see two cases but may see three.

To pass, candidates must usually obtain a mark of 7 or more from the examining team. A borderline mark in one case (e.g., $6\frac{1}{2}$ is a 'fail') may be put up to a pass ($6\frac{1}{2}$ with a 'lift') if all the other cases, including the long case, are above average. One poor performance will usually mean a failure. The examiners do try to be fair. Each candidate's performance is discussed at the end of each long and short case segment and at the end of the day's examining. The written examination mark is not taken into account. On occasions when a candidate is borderline to the point where the four examiners who have seen him or her have been unable to make a final decision, then the candidate will be taken through a separate short case segment by an additional pair of senior examiners, called the 'Extra Team' (ET for short!). This gives the candidate a genuine extra chance. However, they are not trying to pass candidates, as at undergraduate level, but are trying to evaluate the true standard of the candidate. The examinees must prove to the College that they are 'good enough', i.e., they must demonstrate that they have reached the required standard. And the standards are very high!

To achieve uniform standards, the Committee for Examinations has been constantly working on improvements. Senior members of the Committee examine more often with less experienced examiners. The Committee also holds regular formal calibration exercises, in which all the examiners view videotapes and mark a candidate's performance. A general discussion is then held to try to develop a uniformity of approach. There is no doubt that problems continue, as it remains very difficult (if not impossible) to judge ability accurately in such a short period; however, the Committee is working towards eliminating obvious mistakes.

# PREPARATION FOR
# THE CLINICAL EXAMINATION

For most candidates the successful approach to the 'viva' depends upon seeing a large number of long and (particularly) short cases. It is usually too late to start seeing practice cases only after having passed the written examination. Preparation should start several months before at least. To practise for the long case, try to set aside a regular time each week. Most physicians, if approached, are only too willing to test-run candidates. Exposure to many different examiners is desirable—this will help iron out mistakes and provide practice in answering different types of questions. Although most teaching hospitals have a training scheme where practice long cases are examined by consultants or senior registrars, this is not enough. It is difficult to quote numbers, but we believe 30 long cases where different specialists act as examiners represent the bare minimum required for preparation. Remember also that each time a patient is admitted to hospital, practice can be gained in the long case technique—this turns overtime into useful preparation time.

Practice for the short cases is even more important. More examinees fail in these than in the long case. It is valuable to have senior colleagues as well as peers take candidates on these. Travelling to other hospitals to practise is worthwhile, because one has to examine in strange surroundings watched by unfamiliar examiners. It also relieves the boredom somewhat. The best practice examiner is the one who frightens candidates a little, but does not demolish them when they make an error. Make use of all the constructive criticism obtainable. Many candidates practise in pairs too—each person taking turns to be the examiner. Practising being an examiner gives an appreciation of the bad habits which annoy the real examiners.

Equipment is always provided at the hospital where the examination is held. However, it is important to bring the following:

1. A familiar stethoscope which has been used for a long time. Do not buy a newer, fancier stethoscope the day before the test—it takes time to get used to a new instrument.
2. A hand-held eye card—obtainable from OPSM for a moderate charge and essential for cranial nerve or eye examinations (p. 206).
3. A new red-topped hat pin—candidates can buy a plain one and paint the top with nail polish. This is invaluable for visual field testing (p. 206).
4. Paper and pens.

It is debatable whether candidates should bring in their own bag of instruments. Many favour bringing their own ophthalmoscope and pocket torch (with new fresh batteries in both). Others also like to have cotton wool and spatulas, as well as tuning forks (256 and 128 Hertz) and a patella hammer, which is too much to carry in the pockets. This has led to a trend for leather briefcases for all the equipment. However, the occasional difficult examiner has been known to complain about this! There is a story that one candidate's briefcase was filled with such elaborate equipment, including an inverted cardigan for testing dressing apraxia, that his examiners spent their time inspecting the contents rather than watching him examine the patient.

During practice sessions it is a good idea always to place equipment in the same pockets. Candidates do not want to be fumbling at the crucial time—it will only create a poor impression. Consultants carry their stethoscopes or put them in their coat pocket—rarely do they place them around their neck. This seems a sensible policy for aspiring consultants also. A candidate who does carry a briefcase into the test (and many neurologists carry one everywhere) should probably give it to the 'bulldog' whilst doing the short cases. This way the candidate will not run into objections from those examining.

Some candidates take beta-blockers on the day of the test. An interesting story from *Lancet* highlights this very situation. A Scottish physician refers to a British (not an Irish) censor who had the habit of counting the temporal pulse of candidates; if he found the pulse rate was less than 60/minute he would take this fact into account when giving his mark. (Bamber, M.G. Dope test for doctors? *Lancet* 1980;ii:1308.) The authors are unaware of a similar practice in Australasia. It is important for candidates intending to use these drugs to give themselves a dose during a practice session. One doctor learnt, to his horror, that beta-blockers caused him severe bronchospasm only at the actual examination (he failed).

Nervous individuals with a tendency to sweat can have problems. One candidate who was balding and wore glasses found, during times of intense stress, that rivers of sweat rolled down from his forehead to fog up his glasses and wash them from his nose. His solution was antiperspirant (unscented of course) applied to the forehead (he passed).

Dress is important. The medical establishment is well known for its conservatism, and non-verbal communication should not be forgotten when dressing. Traditionally gentlemen wear a conservative suit and a non-committal tie. Other important things are short, tidy hair, a neatly trimmed beard if you cannot bear to shave it off, and a neutral smell. Women should dress formally, with care to project an air of quiet efficiency combined with personal attractiveness. White coats are never worn. However, being well dressed is no guarantee of success. There is a story that two male candidates, wearing grey suits and with recently cut hair, once viewed with satisfaction a third examinee whose long hair was tied neatly in a bun, and whose kaftan and sandals with bells were topped off with a shoulder bag; they felt their own success seemed assured with such competition. However, it turned out that they were unsuccessful, and their informally dressed colleague (who was unusually brilliant) passed.

Preparation is the key to success. Like an Olympic athlete, obtain plenty of sleep in the week before the ordeal; take no alcohol or tranquillizers in the 48 hours before it, and do not study during the final 24. Make sure you eat something on the day of the examination and avoid a long trip to the examination city on the morning or the night before the test.

# Chapter 5

# THE LONG CASE

*The man who confesses his ignorance shows it once;*
*he who tries to conceal it shows it many times.*

Japanese Proverb

When the examiners discuss a long case with a candidate they are expecting to find out how he or she would manage the patient and their problems. They want to know if the candidate has a practical grasp of what is required in consultant practice. Practising long cases trains candidates to be better clinicians.

A careful allocation of time with the patient is vital. The exact proportions will depend on the case itself, but as a rough guide, spend 25 minutes on the history, 20 minutes on the examination, and the rest of the time preparing discussion and reviewing vital facts with the patient. Nothing is more important than leaving enough time to get one's thoughts in order.

People favour many different systems for recording long case details (as an aid to memory). There are two we recommend. One is to use a small pad which can be held comfortably in the hand and the pages turned unobtrusively. The other is a small card system. One side is used for the history, and the other for the examination findings; a second card (if necessary) is used for relevant investigations, management, and short lists of facts the candidate may wish to mention. Obviously numbering of each side is important so as not to mix up the order of presentation. Candidates who do not wish to rewrite the whole long case presentation before facing the examiners (time is often a problem) may find it helpful to number the paragraphs with a red pen in the order they wish to present the story.

Once a candidate has said 'hello' to the patient at the beginning of the long case, we suggest initially following the steps outlined below. These may help the candidate rapidly to ascertain the patient's major problems so that further questioning may be directed more easily.

1. Explain to the patient that this is a very important examination. Gain his or her interest and support. This is a test of bedside manner.
2. Ask the patient what is wrong. If he or she says 'Am I allowed to tell you?',

look confident and firm and say 'Yes, of course'. Candidates are entitled to all the information the patient can offer.

3. Ask why the patient is in hospital this time (i.e., is he or she an inpatient or out-patient?) and, if relevant, the presenting symptoms when the patient was admitted.
4. Ask early what medications the patient is taking. This will give valuable information about both current and past problems.
5. Ask about any recent tests, again to obtain clues about the current problem.

In the majority of long cases, the patient has a chronic illness about which he or she may be very well informed. It is sensible to make use of this knowledge, but remember the trap that patients may be biased in their opinions and give (inadvertently) false information. Having established the main diagnosis early, confirm this with specific questioning. On finding symptoms not fitting the diagnosis, decide the likely possibilities and follow them up with further questions. Never blindly believe the patient.

Enquire about other problems next. Most long case patients are chosen because they have multiple medical problems. An example might be an elderly lady with pulmonary fibrosis as her major presenting illness who also has significant ischaemic heart disease and moderate renal impairment secondary to analgesic abuse. It is a terrible experience to discover another major illness only minutes before the end of the time. List all the important diseases chronologically. Obtain full details about each. Organize to present the most important (i.e., current) problem first, followed by the others in order of importance.

Don't forget the social history. This is especially important as the examiners are keen to have caring specialists who are fully aware of the social environment of their patients.

Always ask about:

*Occupation*—now and in the past.

*Adequacy of income*—particularly if the patient is on the pension.

*Ability to cope* at home and the quality of life if this is a chronic disease problem.

*Mobility*—particularly the number of steps that need to be climbed at home and at work, and on which floor the patient lives.

*Hobbies*.

*Marital status* and number of children.

*Sexual problems*—particularly ask about impotence in males (e.g., in diabetic patients).

*Place of birth*.

*Overseas travel* in relationship to the illness.

This sort of information is easy to obtain, and fills in discussion time neatly, but disaster can threaten if it is not known. A family history must also be taken. Only those areas that are relevant to the presenting problems should be mentioned in the discussion.

As one examines the patient, one should always ask when the examiners came, what parts were examined, and whether any comments were made about the signs.

One candidate was told by his patient that, during a fundoscopy examination, the examiner had said: 'What an interesting Roth's spot!' However, this is no substitute for a thorough examination.

Even though the candidate should spend most time on the relevant systems, remember that sometimes unexpected signs may crop up, such as a large breast mass, gross papilloedema or an abdominal mass. The examiners always have in front of them a list of the signs and have always gone to the trouble of checking that in fact these signs are present. The candidate will be expected to have found all the important signs, so be thorough. Any very equivocal findings should probably be ignored. Ask the 'bulldog' for the results of the urine analysis and the rectal examination. The candidate is not expected to perform these personally. Also, don't forget to take the blood pressure at some stage and check for a postural change, if at all relevant (e.g., diabetes mellitus, p. 199).

At the end of the history taking and the physical examination, always ask: 'Is there anything else you think I should know?' Amazingly important information is often volunteered at this point. Then ask yourself, 'Could this be anything else?' and 'Can I tie all the multisystem problems into one disease?'

During the 20 minutes or so remaining, decide what type of case it is—i.e., is this a MANAGEMENT problem, or a DIAGNOSTIC problem, or both? Draft the introductory statement—e.g., 'I saw Mrs J. Smith, a 50-year-old woman who presents with the management problem of active rheumatoid arthritis, and also the diagnostic and management problem of chronic liver disease.'

Next, mentally rehearse presenting the history and examination concisely and clearly. The concluding statement should reiterate the problems (in order of importance). It is usual to end the presentation by requests for relevant investigations. Always formulate a differential diagnosis, even if the history and examination lead to a positive diagnosis. If a positive diagnosis cannot confidently be made, one should try to decide the most likely diagnosis.

The whole presentation to the examiners should take about seven minutes. Leave out any irrelevant detail—padding the presentation is never impressive. Also remember never to use abbreviations when presenting—e.g., for jugular venous pressure, or metacarpophalangeal joint. The examiners are only human too—sometimes they are hungry, tired, or just bored following previous presentations. Show interest and enthusiasm whilst speaking. Don't read notes in an uninteresting monotone. The notes are meant to be a memory aid. Ideally, the long case should be a discussion between consultants, with the candidate being a respectful junior colleague. The examiners only very occasionally interrupt during the presentation. At the end they may try to clarify a particular point. Sometimes they direct the candidate onto a particular line of discussion.

The discovery of a major problem with a particular long case (e.g., the patient with obvious dementia) shouldn't lead to panic. By recognizing the problem, fully examining the patient, and having a plan of management (finding reversible causes, eliciting from relatives the social setup, etc.), the candidate will pass. One candidate who was faced with a demented patient in the long case examination did become angry and bitterly complained to his examiners. He failed.

Occasionally there can be other difficulties, such as language problems (usually the candidate is supplied with an interpreter, often a relative), or the patient becomes ill during the time (cardiac arrests have occurred). Be sure to inform the 'bulldog' of any difficulties—everyone goes out of his or her way to be fair in such circumstances.

When appropriate, ask for one or two important investigations relevant to the problems, rather than for a string of routine tests. A reason should always be given for ordering the test. Any mentioned test may have to be discussed in detail with the examiners. We suggest that you write down the results you are told—it is embarrassing to have to ask for the figures to be repeated. Don't ignore any information that is given—e.g., if the haemoglobin value is normal, comment on this and explain how it helps. Remember not to touch X-ray films or criticize the quality of the material shown. Pathology specimens are not shown in the clinical examinations.

Always prepare answers to the obvious lines of question. In a management case, for example, prepare an outline of the suggested management and be able to justify it. Theoretical aspects of the condition may be asked about (e.g., the causes of chronic liver disease, or the complement changes in infective endocarditis), so prepare these beforehand.

If the candidate is answering well, the line of questioning may change, or the depth may become overwhelming. Do NOT be frightened to say in the latter situation, 'Sir (or Madam), I don't know' when asked a very difficult question. Obvious wild guesses will be detrimental. If the examiner persists in asking a question, it usually means he or she is trying to establish a very basic fact. Talk sensibly around the topic—often a supplementary question will result in recall of the appropriate information.

You must be able to discuss sensibly anything that you mention in a 'viva', so don't casually allude to diseases that you know nothing about—e.g., kala-azar as a cause of massive splenomegaly.

# Chapter 6

# COMMON LONG CASES

*In what manner are the examiners elected? Are they elected by the profession or any part of the profession whose interests are equal to those of the whole, and are they responsible to the profession at large for their conduct? Neither the one nor the other.*

Lancet 1824;i:205

Important and common long cases are presented in some detail in this section. The list (see Table 6-1) is not exhaustive, but gives an idea of the range of possible cases. Most (but not all) are discussed here—some other relevant aspects are dealt with in the short case chapter.

They are written as a guide to dealing with the long case examination but are not meant to replace textbook descriptions. To pass you must really know and understand your general medicine. Remember that usually several problems occur in the one case.

## INFECTIVE ENDOCARDITIS

Since these patients stay in hospital for weeks, they are often available for long cases. The disease presents both diagnostic, and short and long term management problems. It combines cardiological, microbiological and immunological aspects. The diagnosis is usually known to the patient. An intravenous infusion containing antibiotics is a valuable clue.

### The History

Ask about:

1. Details of presenting symptoms, e.g., malaise, fever, symptoms of anaemia.
2. Symptoms suggesting embolic phenomena to large vessels (e.g., brain, viscera) or small vessels (e.g., kidney with haematuria or loin pain).

**Table 6-1.** *Common Long Cases*

**Cardiovascular System:**
1. Infective Endocarditis (p. 33)
2. Congestive Cardiac Failure (p. 38)
3. Hyperlipidemia (p. 41)
4. Heart Transplantation (p. 44)
5. Valvular Heart Disease (p. 142)

**Respiratory System:**
1. Bronchiectasis (p. 48)
2. Lung Carcinoma (p. 51)
3. Chronic Obstructive Pulmonary Disease (p. 54)
✓4. Pulmonary Fibrosis (p. 56)
5. Sarcoidosis (p. 58)
6. Cystic Fibrosis (p. 61)

**Gastrointestinal System:**
1. Malabsorption (p. 64)
2. Inflammatory Bowel Disease (p. 68)
3. Chronic Liver Disease (p. 72)
4. Liver Transplantation (p. 77)

**Haemopoietic System:**
1. Haemolytic Anaemia (p. 80)
2. Polycythaemia Rubra Vera (p. 82)
3. Lymphoma (p. 87)
4. Multiple Myeloma (p. 90)

**Rheumatology:**
1. Rheumatoid Arthritis (p. 92)
2. Ankylosing Spondylitis (p. 204)
3. Systemic Lupus Erythematosus (p. 97)
4. Scleroderma (p. 102)

**Endocrine:**
1. Thyrotoxicosis (p. 187)
2. Hypothyroidism (p. 188)
3. Panhypopituitarism (p. 189)
4. Cushing's Syndrome (p. 190)
5. Acromegaly (p. 192)
6. Addison's Disease (p. 195)
7. Paget's Disease (p. 105)
8. Diabetes Mellitus (p. 108, 197)

**Renal System:**
1. Chronic Renal Failure (p. 113)
2. Renal Transplantation (p. 119)
3. Nephrotic Syndrome (Table 6-35 p. 114)

**Central Nervous System:**
1. Multiple Sclerosis (p. 122)
2. Myasthenia Gravis (p. 124)
3. Guillain-Barré Syndrome (p. 126)

**Infectious Disease:**
1. Pyrexia of Unkown Origin (PUO) (p. 128)

3. Recent dental or operative procedures—the average time between procedure and diagnosis is 100 days.
4. Use of antibiotics either for prophylaxis before an invasive procedure or for rheumatic fever prophylaxis or both.
5. A past history of rheumatic fever.
6. A history of other heart disease or heart operations, especially of valve replacement.
7. History of intravenous drug abuse, particularly for tricuspid and pulmonary valve infection.
8. Antibiotic allergies.
9. How the diagnosis was made—including the number of blood cultures, and the use of echocardiography.
10. Management since admission to hospital, including the names of the antibiotics used, duration of treatment, and whether the possibility of valve replacement has been discussed.
11. History of other major diseases, particularly those associated with immune suppression, e.g., steroids.

## The Examination (p. 135)

Start by examining for the peripheral stigmata of endocarditis.

1. Hands:
   (a) Clubbing (a late sign)
   (b) Splinter haemorrhages
   (c) Osler's nodes on the finger pulp (probably an embolic phenomenon—these are rare)
   (d) Janeway lesions (non-tender erythematous maculopapular lesions containing bacteria, on the palms or pulps—very rare).
2. Eyes: Roth's spots in the fundus, conjunctival petechiae.
3. Abdomen: Splenomegaly (a late sign).
4. Urine analysis for haematuria and proteinuria.
5. Neurological signs of embolic disease.
6. Joints (occasionally resembles rheumatic fever pattern).

Next examine the heart. Assess for predisposing cardiac lesions. These are in order:

1. Acquired:
   (a) mitral incompetence S
   (b) mitral stenosis D
   (c) aortic stenosis S
   (d) aortic incompetence D
   (e) mitral valve prolapse
2. Congenital:
   (a) bicuspid aortic valve
   (b) patent ductus arteriosus
   (c) ventricular septal defect
   (d) coarctation of the aorta

N.B. Remember an atrial septal defect of the secundum type is almost never affected.

Examine for the signs of cardiac failure. Look for signs of a prosthetic valve (Table 8-4 p. 141) and for scars that may be present from previous valvotomy or repair operations. Look for a source of infection and take the patient's temperature.

## Investigations

1. Three to six blood cultures (at least) over 24 hours (98% of culture-positive cases will give positive results in the first three bottles).
2. Full blood count and erythrocyte sedimentation rate (ESR). Look for anaemia—normochromic, normocytic—neutrophilia and an elevated ESR—which may be greater than 100mm in one hour.
3. Renal function.
4. Chest X-ray film. Look for left-or-right ventricular hypertrophy, increased pulmonary artery markings, Kerley's B lines, frank cardiac failure, valve calcification (lateral film).
5. Electrocardiogram. Atrial fibrillation in the elderly (particularly common) and conduction defects may occur but are not specific.
6. Echocardiography (M mode, 2D and Doppler). Vegetations must be larger than 2mm to be detected. This procedure cannot distinguish active from inactive lesions. Vegetations are seen in approximately 40% of cases. Transoesophageal echocardiography may allow better definition of valvular involvement. Doppler examination may reveal new valvular regurgitation.
7. Serological tests. These include tests for immune complexes, and classical pathway activation of complement causing low $C_3$, low $C_4$, and low CH50 levels. The test for rheumatoid factor gives positive results in 50% of cases and that for antinuclear factor in 20% of cases.

## Notes

### Organisms

1. *Streptococcus viridans* (non-haemolytic) usually presents subacutely.
2. *Streptococcus faecalis*—particularly in old men with prostatism.
3. *Streptococcus bovis*—associated with bowel carcinoma.
4. *Staphylococcus aureus*—particularly in drug addicts; usually presents acutely.
5. *Staphylococcus epidermidis*—more common in patients with recent valve replacement.
6. Gram-negative coccobacilli rarely a cause—most common with prosthetic valves.
7. Fungi (e.g., Candida, Aspergillus)—particularly drug addicts and immunosuppressed patients.

### Causes of Culture-negative Endocarditis

1. Previous use of antibiotics.
2. Exotic organisms, e.g., *Haemophilus parainfluenzae*, histoplasmosis, *Brucella*, monilia, Q fever.
3. Right-sided endocarditis (rarely).

## *Post Valvotomy Endocarditis*

Early infection is acquired at operation; late infection occurs from another source.

# Treatment

1. Intravenous administration of a bactericidal antibiotic. If the organism is a sensitive *Strep. viridans*, give penicillin, 10 000 000 to 20 000 000 units per day, intravenously for two weeks then orally for two weeks. If it is an entero-coccus, at least four weeks of intravenous treatment are necessary and the choice of antibiotic depends on the organism's sensitivity. For prosthetic valves, from six to eight weeks of intravenous treatment is necessary.
2. Follow the progress by looking at the fever chart, serological results, and hae- Hb. moglobin values.
3. Indications for surgery:
   (a) resistant organisms, e.g., fungi
   (b) valvular dysfunction causing moderate to severe cardiac failure, e.g. acute severe aortic incompetence
   (c) persistently positive blood cultures in spite of treatment
   (d) invasive paravalvular infection causing conduction disturbances, or a para-valvular abscess or fistula (detected by echocardiography) Sinus of Valsalva.
   (e) recurrent major embolic phenomena, although this is controversial (an isolated vegetation is not in itself an indication for surgery)
   N.B. Close consultation with a cardiothoracic surgeon is helpful in serious cases, e.g., staphylococcal infections or patients with prosthetic valves.

## *Factors Suggesting a Poorer Prognosis*

1. Shock.
2. Congestive cardiac failure.
3. Extreme age.
4. Aortic valve or multiple valve involvement.
5. Multiple organisms.
6. Culture-negative endocarditis.
7. Delay in starting treatment.
8. Prosthetic valve involvement.
9. Staphylococcal, Gram-negative and fungal infections.

## *Differential Diagnosis*

1. Atrial myxoma.
2. Occult malignant neoplasm.
3. Systemic lupus erythematosus (p. 97).
4. Polyarteritis nodosa.
5. Post-streptococcal glomerulonephritis.
6. Fever of unknown origin (p. 128).

## Prognosis

Prior to antibiotic use, this was an invariably fatal disease; over 70% of patients with endogenous infection now survive, as do 50% of those with a prosthetic valve infection. Intravenous drug users have a good prognosis.

*[handwritten margin note: Amp 2g/Vanc 1g / Gent 120mg / Rpt / after 8 hrs]*

## Prophylaxis

Confusion about rheumatic fever and endocarditis prophylaxis is rife. Rheumatic fever prophylaxis consists of long-term, low-dose antibiotic administration. Prophylaxis against endocarditis requires high-dose, short-term treatment in any patient with a prosthetic heart valve, congenital heart malformation, acquired valve disease, surgically constructed pulmonary shunt, hypertrophic cardiomyopathy, or a past history of endocarditis.

Prophylaxis regimens are as follows (American Heart Association recommendations):

*[handwritten margin note: Penicillin V / 2g before / 1g 6° after / Erythromycin / 1g 1° before / 500mg 6° after]*

1. *Dental procedures* (e.g., gum cleaning) or oral surgery—Penicillin V (2g) one hour before the procedure, followed by 1g six hours later. If the risk is high (e.g., prosthetic valve), give ampicillin and gentamicin as described below. For those allergic to penicillin, 1g of erythromycin, given orally one hour before the procedure, followed by 500mg six hours later, is adequate.
2. *Enterococcal risk* (e.g., cystoscopy)
   Ampicillin 2g plus gentamicin 1.5mg/kg by intramuscular or intravenous injection half an hour before the procedure, and repeat this eight hours later. For those allergic to penicillin, vancomycin 1g plus gentamicin is adequate.

# CONGESTIVE CARDIAC FAILURE

This is a common therapeutic problem. It may be a diagnostic problem. It is uncommonly the only major problem in a long case in the examination.

## The History

1. It is important first to find out what has precipitated the patient's admission to hospital, and for how long he or she has been in hospital. Precipitating problems include:
   (a) arrhythmias;
   (b) discontinuation of medications (particularly important);
   (c) anaemia;
   (d) infection and fever;
   (e) myocardial infarction;
   (f) pregnancy;
   (g) thyrotoxicosis (p. 187);
   (h) sudden hypotension;

**Table 6-2.** *Causes of Ventricular Failure*

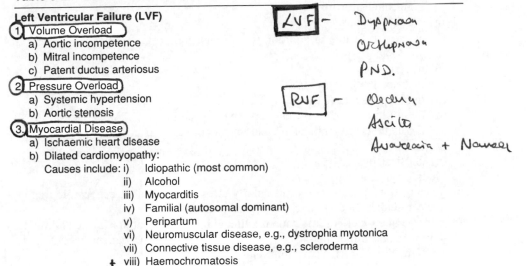

**Left Ventricular Failure (LVF)**

1. Volume Overload
   - a) Aortic incompetence
   - b) Mitral incompetence
   - c) Patent ductus arteriosus
2. Pressure Overload
   - a) Systemic hypertension
   - b) Aortic stenosis
3. Myocardial Disease
   - a) Ischaemic heart disease
   - b) Dilated cardiomyopathy:
     - Causes include:
       - i) Idiopathic (most common)
       - ii) Alcohol
       - iii) Myocarditis
       - iv) Familial (autosomal dominant)
       - v) Peripartum
       - vi) Neuromuscular disease, e.g., dystrophia myotonica
       - vii) Connective tissue disease, e.g., scleroderma
       - viii) Haemochromatosis
       - ix) Sarcoidosis
       - x) Drugs, e.g., doxorubicin
       - xi) Radiation
       - xii) Diabetes mellitus

N.B. Restrictive cardiomyopathy and hypertrophic cardiomyopathy (p. 153) can be causes of heart failure also.

**Right Ventricular Failure (RVF)**

1. Volume Overload
   - a) Atrial septal defect
   - b) Tricuspid incompetence
2. Pressure Overload
   - a) Pulmonary stenosis
   - b) Pulmonary hypertension
3. Myocardial Disease
   - a) Cardiomyopathy secondary to left ventricular failure

(handwritten: LVF — Dyspnoea, Orthopnoea, PND. RVF — Oedema, Ascites, Anorexia + Nausea; Pulmonary embolism)

 

(i) pulmonary embolism;

(j) high salt intake, or excessive physical exertion.

N.B. Chronic lung disease can be a cause of, or a precipitating factor for right and left ventricular failure (p. 54).

2. Then ask about the symptoms of left ventricular failure (e.g., dyspnoea, orthopnoea, paroxysmal nocturnal dyspnoea) and right ventricular failure (e.g., oedema, ascites, anorexia and nausea). Ask about symptoms of ischaemic heart disease (e.g., angina).

3. History of previous heart disease:
   (a) hypertension;

    (b) ischaemic heart disease—infarcts, angina;
    (c) rheumatic or other valve disease;
    (d) congenital heart disease;
    (e) cardiomyopathy.
4. Coronary risk factors in addition to age and male sex:
    (a) smoking;
    (b) hypertension;
    (c) diabetes mellitus (p. 108);
    (d) hyperlipidaemia (p. 41);
    (e) family history of early coronary heart disease;
    (f) the contraceptive pill or premature menopause;
    (g) obesity;
    (h) physical inactivity.
5. Medications currently taken.
6. Investigations undertaken—particularly stress ECG testing, echocardiography, nuclear studies, and cardiac catheterization.
7. How the disease affects the patient's life, ability to cope at home (e.g., climbing stairs), sexual difficulties, etc. Remember to classify the patient according to the New York Heart Association class:

    I    angina/dyspnoea on more than usual activity;
    II   angina/dyspnoea on usual activity;
    III  angina/dyspnoea on less than ordinary activity;
    IV  angina/dyspnoea at rest.

## The Examination (p. 135)

Perform a detailed cardiovascular system examination. Particularly look for signs of cardiac failure, the underlying causes of the problem, and any precipitating factors.

## Investigations

1. Chest X-ray film. Look for cardiomegaly and chamber size (e.g., left atrium), cardiac aneurysm, valve calcification, lung disease, and pulmonary congestion (pp. 148, 149).
2. Electrocardiogram. Look for arrhythmias, signs of ischaemia or recent infarction, left ventricular hypertrophy, and pericarditis.
3. Electrolytes and creatinine levels to exclude hypokalaemia (as a cause of arrhythmia), hyponatraemia (which may indicate severe long-standing cardiac failure, a poor prognostic sign), and renal failure.
4. Haemoglobin value. Exclude anaemia as a precipitating cause.
5. If the diagnosis is not already obvious, consider dilated cardiomyopathy. Investigations for this include:

    (a) Echocardiography which will show generalized poor contractility and reduced fractional shortening.

(b) A gated blood pool scan for the ejection fraction.

(c) Coronary angiography which is often necessary to exclude coronary artery disease. If appropriate, evaluate for the causes of dilated cardiomyopathy.

(d) Right ventricular biopsy may help determine the aetiology in selected patients.

## Treatment

1. Remove precipitating causes.
2. Correct underlying causes if possible (table 6-2).
3. Control the failure:

(a) Decrease physical activity, e.g., avoid exertion to the point of breathlessness, bed rest.

(b) Increase myocardial contractility, e.g., with digoxin.

N.B. The use of digoxin in cardiac failure is controversial. Patients most likely to benefit have more severe heart failure, an S-3 gallop, impressive cardiomegaly, and an ejection fraction less than 20%. Many cardiologists do not consider it useful in the presence of sinus rhythm.

(c) Control fluid retention, e.g., by low-salt diet, fluid restriction, diuretics.

(d) Reduce preload and afterload. Long-acting nitrates are useful venodilators. Angiotensin converting enzyme (ACE) inhibitors are considered by some to be the drug class of choice as they prolong life; hypotension is the major side effect in cardiac failure. The combination of nitrates and hydralazine also improves the prognosis and should be considered in patients unable to take ACE inhibitors.

(e) Intravenous inotropes (e.g., dopamine or dobutamine) may have a place in the short-term treatment of severe cardiac failure.

Cardiac transplantation may now be offered to certain patients (see p. 44).

# HYPERLIPIDAEMIA

Hyperlipidaemia may be present in patients admitted to hospital for the investigation of vascular disease, pancreatitis, hypothyroidism, or diabetes mellitus. They often present both diagnostic and management problems.

## The History

1. The patient should be able to indicate whether the main problem is vascular or not. If the problem is one of premature coronary artery disease, hypercholesterolaemia is the likely lipid problem. The most important inherited cause is *familial hypercholesterolaemia*, which is caused by a defective or absent low density lipoprotein (LDL) receptor. The heterozygous form occurs in about one person in five hundred. Since the transmission is autosomal dominant, the patient may know of first degree relatives who have been affected. There may even be

family members with the homozygous form. These people usually present with a tenfold elevation in serum cholesterol due to an increase in plasma LDL, and have a myocardial infarction before the age of 20 years. People with the heterozygous form typically have myocardial infarctions in their 30s and 40s and have a twofold to threefold elevation in cholesterol. Over 80% of affected males and nearly 60% of affected females have had myocardial infarcts by the age of 60 years. Find out if the patient has already had a myocardial infarct and which of his or her relatives has been affected.

*Familial combined hyperlipidaemia* is associated with obesity or glucose intolerance and may be expressed as type IIa, IIb, or IV hyperlipidemia (Table 6-3). This is also an autosomal dominant trait. Patients develop hypercholesterolaemia and often hypertriglyceridaemia in puberty. Once again there usually is a strong family history of premature coronary artery disease.

*Familial dysbetalipoproteinaemia* is also associated with coronary artery disease. These patients have elevated cholesterol and triglyceride levels and are usually found to have obesity, hypothyroidism or diabetes mellitus. Find out whether there is any history of these and whether there has been atheromatous disease or vascular disease involving the internal carotid arteries and abdominal aorta or its branches.

Ask about claudication, which occurs in about one-third of patients.

2. The patient may be able to tell you his or her cholesterol and triglyceride levels and what they have been in the past.

3. If there is no history of coronary disease and the patient either knows the triglyceride level to have been very high, or has a history of pancreatitis, the likely diagnosis is *familial hypertriglyceridaemia*. This is also a common autosomal dominant disorder and is associated with obesity, hyperglycaemia, hyperinsulinaemia, hypertension, and hyperuricaemia. Although there is a slightly increased incidence of atherosclerosis, this is probably related to diabetes, obesity and hypertension rather than to the hypertriglyceridaemia itself.

Ask about the patient's alcohol consumption or any history of hypothyroidism or the ingestion of oestrogen-containing contraceptive pills. Any of these can precipitate a rapid rise in the triglyceride level which may precipitate pancreatitis or the characteristic eruptive xanthomas. In between attacks patients have moderate elevations of the plasma triglyceride level.

4. Next find out about treatment. In familial hypercholesterolaemia this will have been aimed at the cholesterol level itself and at any cardiovascular complications that have occurred. The patient should be well informed about a low cholesterol diet and may be aware of side effects from medication usage.

Treatment is usually begun with one of the bile sequestering resins—cholestyramine or colestipol. These bind bile salts in the gut so that cholesterol is withdrawn from the circulation by the liver to make more. They are not absorbed but can cause constipation, flatulence, and block the absorption of other drugs. The patient may need to take up to two sachets three times daily. If the cholesterol cannot be brought down to normal levels with diet and a resin, nicotinic acid which blocks very low density lipoprotein (VLDL) synthesis may have been added. This is quite an effective drug and may help block the compensating increase in hepatic cholesterol synthesis that occurs with bile sequestering resins. Side effects include flushing, pruritis, abnormal liver function test results, hyperglycaemia, and aggravation of peptic ulcer disease. The patient will probably have been begun on a small dose and had this gradually increased as tolerance improves.

Some patients may be taking HMG CoA reductase inhibitors (e.g., lovastatin). These work by inhibiting synthesis of cholesterol in the liver by impeding the activity of the rate-limiting enzyme. Patients need to have their liver function monitored monthly and have yearly ophthalmological checks for lens opacities. Gemfibrozil increases the activity of lipoprotein lipase and is useful in hypertrigylceridaemia due to increased VLDL or intermediate density lipoproteins (IDL); clofibrate is no longer in common use for lipid control.

Patients with homozygous familial hypercholesterolaemia are unlikely to live long enough to be present in exams but treatment for these people can sometimes involve repeated plasma exchange and even liver transplantation.

A patient with one of the combined hyperlipidaemias is likely to need to lose weight as well as control the cholesterol and saturated fat intake, and with dysbetalipoproteinaemia may require treatment for hypothyroidism. All these patients need to avoid alcohol and the oral contraceptive pill. Diet is the mainstay of treatment for reducing triglyceride levels; gemfibrozil may be used if diet fails.

A patient with familial hypertriglyceridaemia will have been treated in a similar way and may have required treatment for acute pancreatitis.

## The Examination (p. 135)

Examine the cardiovascular system where there may be evidence of cardiac failure from previous myocardial infarcts.

Look specifically for the interesting skin manifestations of these conditions. Patients with the heterozygous form of familial hypercholesterolaemia have tendon xanthomas. These are nodular swellings which tend to involve the tendons of the knee, elbow, dorsum of the hand, and the achilles tendon. They consist of massive deposits of cholesterol, probably derived from the deposition of LDL particles. They contain both amorphous extracellular deposits and vacuoles within macrophages. Cholesterol deposits in the soft tissue of the eyelid cause xanthelasma and those in the cornea produce arcus cornea. The tendon xanthomas are diagnostic of familial hypercholesterolaemia but the other signs are not so specific. Up to three-quarters of patients with the heterozygous form have these signs.

Patients with the homozygous form have even more interesting signs. Yellow xanthomas occur at points of trauma and in the webs of the fingers. Tendon xanthomas, arcus cornea and xanthelasma also occur. Cholesterol deposits in the aortic valve may be sufficient to cause aortic stenosis; occasionally mitral stenosis and mitral regurgitation can occur for the same reason. Painful swollen joints may also be present. Obesity is uncommon in these patients.

If the history suggests combined hyperlipidaemia or hypertriglyceridaemia, obesity is likely to be present. Look also for signs of the complications of diabetes mellitus (p. 108), and for signs of hypothyroidism (p. 188) or the nephrotic syndrome (p. 114). Examine the abdomen for tenderness as an indication of pancreatitis.

## Investigations

A cholesterol level over 8mmol/L with a normal triglyceride level suggests familial hyperlipidaemia. The diagnosis can be confirmed by an assay of the number of LDL receptors on blood lymphocytes. The diagnosis is more often made from a combination of the lipid pattern, the history, and the clinical examination (Table 6-3). The other necessary investigations are those required for coronary artery disease.

Investigation of hypertriglyceridaemia includes tests to exclude possible under-lying causes including hypothyroidism, diabetes mellitus, and excessive alcohol intake. In familial hypertriglyceridaemia the plasma triglyceride level tends to be moderately elevated—3 to 6mmol/L (type IV lipoprotein pattern). The cholesterol level is normal. The triglyceride level may rise to values in excess of 12mmol/L during exacerbations of the condition.

Familial combined hyperlipidaemia produces one of three different lipoprotein patterns—hypercholesterolaemia (type IIa), hypertriglyceridaemia (type IV) or both hypercholesterolaemia and hypertriglyceridaemia.

Familial dysbetalipoproteinaemia (type III hyperlipoproteinaemia) results in the accumulation of large lipoprotein particles containing triglycerides and choles-terol. These particles resemble the remnants and IDL particles normally produced from the catabolism of chylomicrons and VLDL. The patients have an abnormal apoprotein E which is unable to bind to hepatic lipoprotein receptors, preventing the rapid hepatic uptake of IDL and chylomicrons. The condition is usually only expressed in patients with hypothyroidism or diabetes mellitus and tests for these conditions are necessary.

## Management

A combination of diet and treatment of the underlying condition is usually required (p. 42). Underlying diabetes mellitus and hypothyroidism must be treated. Some patients with dysbetalipoproteinaemia respond dramatically to the introduction of thyroxine. Effective management of the condition tends to cause disappearance of the skin signs and improves the prognosis as far as vascular disease goes. Effective treament of familial hyperlipidaemia from early adult life delays the onset of coronary artery disease.

# HEART TRANSPLANTATION

Cardiac transplantation is now an accepted form of treament for intractable cardiac failure. Increasing numbers of patients who have either had a transplant or are on the waiting list for one are available for clinical exams. Those awaiting transplant are sick enough to require frequent admissions to hospital and those who have had

**Table 6-3.** *Hyperlipoproteinaemias*

| Type | Lipoprotein Elevated | Electro-phoretic Mobility | Mechanism | Secondary Causes | Clinical Features | Associations |
|------|----------------------|---------------------------|-----------|------------------|-------------------|--------------|
| I | Chylomicrons | Origin | Deficiency extrahepatic lipoprotein lipase or apo C-II deficiency | Rarely SLE | Eruptive xanthomata; Lipaemia retinalis | Pancreatitis |
| IIa | LDL | β | Receptor defect | Cushing's; hypothyroidism; cholestasis; nephrotic syndrome | Xanthelasma; Corneal arcus; Tendon xanthomata | CAD, PVD |
| IIb | LDL & VLDL | β & pre-β | | | | |
| III | IDL | Broad β | Oversynthesis and/or abnormal apo E | Renal and liver disease | Palmar crease and tubo-eruptive xanthomata; xanthelasma | CAD, PVD |
| IV | VLDL | Pre-β | Oversynthesis and/or under-catabolism of VLDL | Diabetes mellitus; alcoholism; chronic renal failure | Usually no xanthomata | |
| V | VLDL & chylomicrons | Origin and pre-β | Saturation lipoprotein lipase by VLDL | As for IV | As for I | As for I |

Note:
• apo A-1 deficiency is associated with the absence of plasma HDL and severe premature CAD.
• apo B deficiency is the defect in abetalipoproteinaemia (autosomal recessive) characterized by haemolytic anaemia (acanthocytosis), fat malabsorption and neurological defects (proprioceptive loss, retinitis pigmentosa).
• LCAT deficiency results in decreased HDL, cloudy corneas and progressive renal disease.

LDL = low density lipoprotein; VLDL = very low density lipoprotein; IDL = intemediate density lipoprotein; HDL = high density lipoprotein; CAD = coronary artery disease; PVD = peripheral vascular disease; SLE = systemic lupus erythematosus; apo = apoprotein; LCAT = lecithin cholesterol acyltransferase.

a transplant are often readmitted for various routine investigations. Patients are usually very well informed about their condition and should be able to supply a lot of useful information to the candidate.

Although this fact should not be discussed with our surgical colleagues, heart transplantation is technically not a very difficult operation. Improvements in prognosis have followed medical advances, particularly in the area of the management of rejection. Five-year survival is now slightly over 50% for patients who have received a transplant since 1981, and one-year survival is currently well over 80%.

The examiners will expect a candidate to be familiar with the indications for, and contraindications to the procedure. It is also important to know what investigations are required before a patient can be accepted for surgery and to understand the management problems that can occur in patients who have had the operation (Table 6-4).

## The History

1. Try to establish the cause of the patient's cardiac failure. In younger patients cardiomyopathy is more likely to be the problem but nearly half of patients currently undergoing heart transplant have ischaemic heart disease. Rheumatic valvular heart disease can also affect a younger patient and combined heart and lung transplant is occasionally carried out for patients with primary pulmonary hypertension or cystic fibrosis (p. 61).

    Ask about previous myocardial infarction or angina and whether the patient knows the results of a cardiac catheterization. All patients undergoing a transplant are required to have cardiac catheterization. There may have been a cardiac biopsy performed preoperatively and the patient may be aware of the results of this test. Also ask about previous thoracotomy.

2. Ask about the patient's symptoms before surgery. Get an idea of exercise tolerance and severity of angina if present. The patient may know the results of investigations of cardiac function like exercise tests and gated blood pool scans.

3. Ask what treatment the patient was receiving before transplant—particularly the doses of diuretics and ACE inhibitors. Find out whether frequent admissions to hospital were necessary and whether intravenous inotropes had been required.

4. Find out how long it is since a transplant was performed or how long the patient has been on the waiting list. Ask whether there were any problems with the surgery—either technical or involving acute rejection. Find out how long the patient was in hospital and what further admissions to hospital have occurred since the operation. Ask if a permanent pacemaker was inserted.

5. Endomyocardial biopsies are fairly memorable events and the patient should be able to tell you how frequently these have been performed and when the last one was obtained. It is now routine to carry these out at weekly intervals for the first three weeks postoperatively, every two weeks for the following month, and every six months after that for patients who are stable.

6. Find out what drugs the patient is taking currently. Patients should not require anti-failure treatment but will, of course, be taking immunosuppressive drugs. Almost all patients are now maintained on cyclosporin, whose dose is determined by its serum level, and prednisone. Often azathioprine is also used, and the dose is adjusted according to the white cell count. Sometimes antithymocyte globulin is used early on in treatment or at the onset of a rejection episode. The patient may know of boosts of prednisone that have been given for rejection episodes. Inquire about complications of immunosuppression (p. 79).

7. Some general questions about the patient's current life are very relevant. Find out how much improvement has occurred in the patient's exercise tolerance and whether he or she has been able to go back to work. If the patient is currently an in-patient, find out why he or she has been admitted to hospital on this occasion. Ask about the patient's family and how they have coped with the illness and the transplant itself. Make some discreet inquiries about the patient's finances and whether there have been any problems returning to the transplant hospital for the various investigations that are required.

8. Ask about routine cardiac catheterization. This is performed annually in most patients who have had transplants. Coronary artery intimal proliferation can cause ischaemic heart disease in the transplanted heart. Because the heart has been denervated there is not usually any pain. This intimal proliferation may represent a rejection phenomenon but it is important that the patient's cholesterol be kept as low as possible. Find out if he or she knows what the cholesterol level is and what treatment is being used to keep it low.

## Examination (p. 135)

1. If the transplant has been successful there should not be many signs. A large median sternotomy scar will be present.

2. Look for signs of cardiac failure and pericarditis. Pericarditis can be an indication of rejection.

3. Note the small scars in the neck at the point of introduction of the endomyocardial biopsy forceps.

4. Look for any evidence of Cushing's syndrome from steroid therapy (p. 190).

5. Examine the chest carefully for signs of infection, examine the mouth for candidiasis, look for infection at intravenous sites and look at the temperature chart.

## Investigations

1. These depend somewhat on the reason the patient has been admitted to hospital on this occasion. As mentioned above endomyocardial biopsies are performed routinely and at any suggestion of rejection. Ask about the results of these.

2. A full blood count may be indicated because of possible infection and to monitor the azathioprine dose.

3. Chest X-ray may show signs of cardiac enlargement, though this is a late sign of rejection. Changes on the ECG of rejection include reduction in voltages caused by myocardial oedema, or atrial arrhythmias. Sometimes the patient's ECG shows two sets of P-waves; one comes from the transplanted heart and one arises from the residual atrium.

4. Recent assessments of myocardial function including gated blood pool scans and echocardiograms may be available.

5. Routine coronary angiography may have been performed.
6. If there have been problems with possible infection, results of blood, urine, and other cultures should be sought.

## Management

The discussion should revolve around the patient's current reason for admission. However, there is likely to be time to discuss the management of rejection, infection, cardiac failure or social problems.

1. Rejection. Rejection may have been suspected or diagnosed because of pleuritic chest pain, deterioration in left ventricular function or ECG changes. It is usually diagnosed on the basis of a routine biopsy. The usual approach is to give the patient a boost of methylprednisolone—usually 1g intravenously daily for 3 days followed by a repeat biopsy.
2. Infections occurring as a result of immunosuppression are a major cause of death. Possible episodes of infection should be investigated thoroughly and treated aggressively with appropriate therapy.
3. Further cardiac failure may be an indication of rejection which should be treated. Cardiac failure may also be an indication of silent myocardial infarction.
4. Hyperlipidaemia should be sought routinely and treated most vigorously with drugs and diet.

The discussion of a patient awaiting cardiac transplant will probably run along similar lines. However, it is important to determine how well informed the patient is about what is likely to happen and whether he or she appears to fulfil the criteria for transplantation (Table 6-4).

# BRONCHIECTASIS

This is a fairly common subject for a long case, and usually poses a management problem. Bronchiectasis is defined as pathological dilatation of the bronchi.

## The History

1. Find out when the patient's respiratory problems began. Classically the cough and sputum begin in childhood, though adult onset is becoming more common. The differential diagnosis of cough and sputum since childhood includes cystic fibrosis, tuberculosis, immunoglobulin deficiency, immotile cilia syndrome and asthma. Other symptoms include:
   (a) recurrent haemoptysis;
   (b) dyspnoea and wheeze;
   (c) chronic sinusitis (70%);
   (d) recurrent pneumonia and pleurisy;
   (e) symptoms of right heart failure—a terminal event;
   (f) systemic symptoms of weight loss, fever and anorexia.

**Table 6-4.** *Evaluation for Heart Transplantation*

1. History and examination
2. Body weight
3. Cardiac assessment
    a) Ejection fraction: estimated by resting gated blood pool scan
    b) Echocardiogram: with measurement of left ventricular dimensions and assessment of the cardiac valves. Examination for left ventricular thrombus
    c) Coronary angiography in patients with ischaemic heart disease
    d) 24-hour Holter monitoring to evaluate for ventricular arrhythmias
    e) Right heart catheterization to measure pulmonary vascular resistance and its response to vasodilators. Fixed pulmonary hypertension is a contraindication to cardiac transplantation.
4. HLA tissue typing
5. Chest X-ray and respiratory function tests if indicated
6. Full blood count, ESR and coagulation studies
7. Biochemical profile including liver function tests, electrolytes and estimation of creatinine clearance. Serum cholesterol, triglycerides and blood sugar levels.
8. Serology for antinuclear antibodies and an immunoelectrophoresis
9. Bacteriology. Swabs for methicillin-resistant *Staphylococcus aureus* and a Mantoux test if indicated. Hepatitis A and B, toxoplasma, CMV, EBV, HIV and Herpes simplex serology
10. Psychiatric, renal and dental consultations if required
11. Social work report

If the cause of the cardiomyopathy is unknown, a myocardial biopsy, viral titres (including coxsackie A, echovirus, adeno and influenza titres) and serum iron and total iron binding capacity (for haemochromotosis) are required.

Contraindications for heart transplantation include alcoholism, chronic renal disease, pulmonary parenchymal disease, continued tobacco use, advanced liver disease and advanced age. Diabetes mellitus is a relative contraindication.

ESR = Erythrocyte sedimentation rate; CMV = cytomegalovirus; EBV = Ebstein Barr virus; HIV = human immunodeficiency virus.

2. Recent precipitating cause of admission to hospital, e.g., infection, haemoptysis.
3. Treatment—physiotherapy, postural drainage, antibiotics (as prophylaxis or treatment), bronchodilators, lung resection.
4. Investigations in the past, e.g., CT scanning, bronchograms (memorable!).
5. Aetiology, e.g., childhood or early adult infections (pneumonia, measles, whooping cough) (Table 6-5).
6. How the disease interferes with the patient's quality of life, e.g., work, etc.

## The Examination (p. 160)

Examine the respiratory system carefully. Particularly note the unpleasant purulent sputum and examine carefully for clubbing and localized crackles. Look also for the position of the apex beat (e.g., don't miss dextrocardia) and for the signs of right heart failure. Consider the complications and look for them. These include:

**Table 6-5.** *Causes of Bronchiectasis*

1. Congenital:
    a) Cystic fibrosis
    b) Immotile cilia syndrome
    c) Congenital hypogammaglobulinaemia (especially IgA and IgG subclasses)
2. Acquired:
    a) Infections in childhood, e.g., pneumonia, measles, whooping cough
    b) Localized disease, e.g., bronchial adenoma, tuberculosis, foreign body
    c) Allergic bronchopulmonary aspergillosis (proximal bronchiectasis)

N.B. Lung carcinoma rarely causes bronchiectasis, as death tends to intervene first.

i)    pneumonia;
ii)   pleurisy;
iii)  empyema;
iv)   lung abscess;
v)    cor pulmonale;
vi)   cerebral abscess (very rare);
vii)  amyloid (rate, but an important topic in the examination).

## Investigations

Investigations should include a chest X-ray film (p. 170). This may be normal. It may show 1 to 2cm cystic lesions or, more often, streaky infiltration and thickened bronchial walls, especially in the lower lobes.

Look at the sputum microscopy slide. The common organisms are *Haemophilus influenzae*, *Pseudomonas*, *Escherichia coli*, pneumococcus and *Staphylococcus aureus*. Eosinophilia may indicate aspergillosis or asthma. Ventilatory function tests may show a restrictive defect or an obstructive pattern. Arterial blood gas estimations may show mild or moderate hypoxia and, later, respiratory failure— defined as an arterial $PO_2$ less than 8kPa (60mmHg) or an arterial $PCO_2$ greater than 6.67kPa (50mmHg). Thin section CT scanning of the chest, which is replacing bronchography at many centres, is indicated in young patients to confirm the diagnosis. The disease is usually generalized. If the bronchiectasis is localized, resection may be indicated.

## Treatment

Treatment consists of twice-daily postural drainage (20 minutes morning and night), antibiotics during exacerbations (prophylactic antibiotics are controversial, as are nebulized antibiotics), and bronchodilators to relieve airways obstruction; influenza vaccine is advisable. Management of exacerbations requires more aggressive treatment along similar lines. Treatment of heart failure should go *pari passu* with that of the lung disease. Immunoglobulin deficiency can be treated with monthly intravenous immunoglobulin injections which decrease the incidence of infection and the need for hospitalization. Massive haemoptysis may occur in cystic fibrosis and may respond to bronchial artery embolization. Stopping smoking is always essential.

# LUNG CARCINOMA

This is a common disease which candidates often encounter in the examination. It can pose a diagnostic and management problem. Lung carcinoma remains a leading cause of cancer death in men and women. At diagnosis only 20% will have local disease.

## The History

Ask about:

1. Duration of illness and respiratory symptoms, e.g., haemoptysis, dyspnoea, increasing cough.
2. History of unresolved pneumonia, pleural effusion, or lung abscess.
3. Systemic symptoms (e.g., weight loss).
4. Metastatic and non-metastatic symptoms (Table 6-6).
5. Aetiology:
   (a) Smoking (a dose-response effect—long-term smokers have a risk 20 times increased; discontinuation of smoking reduces the risk over 10 to 15 years but the relative risk does not return to 1.0).
   (b) Occupational history, e.g., asbestos exposure, uranium miners. Remember the effect of asbestos plus smoking is synergistic, *not* additive.
   (c) Chronic scarring, e.g., tuberculosis, scleroderma, pulmonary fibrosis— associated with adenocarcinoma.
6. Investigations performed, e.g., chest X-ray changes (the only abnormal finding in 5% of cases), bronchoscopy, sputum cytology, needle biopsy, thoracotomy.
7. Work and home environment, including the number of dependents.
8. Treatment offered and begun.

## The Examination (p. 160)

Finger clubbing is a most important sign (see Table 8-10, p. 162). This is very rare in small-cell carcinoma. Chest signs will vary—listen carefully for a fixed inspiratory wheeze over a large bronchus. Look for the metastatic and non-metastatic manifestations (especially the neurological and endocrine changes) (Table 6-6).

## Management

Diagnosis may be a problem. Sputum cytology may be helpful in centrally located lesions. The chest X-ray may suggest the cell type, e.g., peripheral nodule

**Table 6-6.** *Metastatic and Non-metastatic Manifestations of Lung Carcinoma*

**Local Extension**
1. Pleural effusion
2. Rib involvement
3. Nerve involvement, e.g., Pancoast's tumour, Horner's syndrome (p. 209), recurrent laryngeal nerve palsy, diaphragmatic paralysis
4. Superior vena caval obstruction (p. 159)
5. Pericardial effusion
6. Oesophageal obstruction
7. Tracheal obstruction
8. Lymphangitis

**Distant Metastases**
1. Cervical adenopathy
2. Cerebral, liver or bone metastases

**Non-Metastatic Features**
1. Anorexia, weight loss, cachexia, fever
2. Endocrine:
   a) hypercalcaemia (increased parathyroid hormone secretion occurs usually in squamous cell carcinoma)
   b) hyponatraemia (antidiuretic hormone—small cell carcinoma)
   c) ectopic ACTH syndrome (usually small cell carcinoma)
   d) gynaecomastia (all types-due to ectopic gonadotrophin secretion)
   e) carcinoid syndrome (small cell carcinoma)
   f) insulin-like activity (squamous cell carcinoma)
3. Skeletal (very rare with small cell carcinoma):
   a) clubbing
   b) hypertrophic pulmonary osteoarthropathy (may be more common with adenocarcinoma)
4. Neurological:
   a) Eaton Lambert's syndrome (small cell carcinoma) (p. 126)
   b) peripheral neuropathy (p. 234) or autonomic neuropathy (p. 199)
   c) subacute cerebellar degeneration (p. 245)
   d) polymyositis/dermatomyositis
   e) cortical degeneration with dementia (p. 222)
   f) acute transverse myelopathy (p. 239)
5. Haematological:
   a) migrating venous thrombophlebitis, arterial thrombosis
   b) diffuse intravascular coagulation
   c) anaemia, leucoerythroblastosis, red cell aplasia, polycythaemia, eosinophilia
6. Skin:
   e.g., acanthosis nigricans (p. 192), fibrinolytic purpura, scleroderma (alveolar cell carcinoma)
7. Renal:
   e.g., nephrotic syndrome (due to membranous glomerulonephritis) (p. 114)
8. Opportunistic Infections (most often in those treated with chemotherapy)

(adenocarcinoma), central lesion with obstructive pneumonitis (squamous), medias-tinal or hilar mass (small cell), or alveolar infiltrate (bronchoalveolar cell). An abnormal shadow on the chest X-ray film should be investigated by flexible fibre-optic bronchoscopy and biopsy. Bronchial brushings and washings should also be sent for cytological examination but have a lower yield than biopsy. For peripheral lesions, especially those less than 2cm in size, transthoracic needle biopsy with CT guidance is useful but complications (e.g., pneumothorax, significant bleeding) are more common. In patients with a malignant pleural effusion, thoracocentesis and pleural biopsy provide a high diagnostic yield (p. 163). Other investigations may need to include bone marrow biopsy, mediastinoscopy and thoracotomy. Other possible causes (e.g., of a coin lesion) must be excluded. For this purpose tomograms are helpful; demonstration of central or lamellar calcification usually indicates that a coin lesion is benign.

Once the diagnosis is made and the cell type is identified, further investigations may be indicated to stage the disease. Symptoms and signs which suggest central nervous system, liver, bone, chest wall, or mediastinal involvement need to be carefully sought. Blood count, serum calcium and liver function tests may suggest tumour spread. CT scan with contrast of the chest and abdomen is an important aid in determining whether disease is localized. In small cell carcinoma, stage the disease into (i) limited disease (lung primary, ipsilateral and contralateral hilar, mediastinal and supraclavicular nodes) or (ii) extensive disease (contralateral lung, distant metastases).

Assessment for resectability should include respiratory function tests; if the $FEV_1$ is 2L or more, this indicates the patient could tolerate a pneumonectomy (an $FEV_1$ postoperatively of 800mL or more is considered necessary).

## Treatment

Small cell carcinomas are rarely resected as they have usually metastasized at the time of diagnosis. In limited disease, chemotherapy and concurrent radiotherapy improve the prognosis. Treatment often includes etoposide and cisplatin. Prophy-lactic cranial irradiation is given to patients with complete responses. There is a risk of leukaemia, central nervous system metastases, dementia, and second pri-mary malignancies with treatment. Limited small-cell carcinoma has a median survival with treatment of 11 to 18 months; 10% to 20% are disease-free at 2 years. Extensive small-cell carcinoma has a median survival of 6 to 12 months with therapy.

Non-small cell carcinomas may be resectable unless there is tumour spread to the contralateral lung or outside the thorax, or there is significant cardiopulmon-ary disease. The most important prognostic factor is the stage of disease. Median survival is only a few months in patients with intracranial metastases or bone involvement.

Airway obstruction due to carcinoma may be relieved by using Nd-YAG laser for palliation.

# CHRONIC OBSTRUCTIVE PULMONARY DISEASE (CHRONIC AIRFLOW LIMITATION)

This general term is usually applied to patients with chronic bronchitis and emphysema. The condition is common and presents major management problems. However, in the examination, it is unusual for it to be the patient's only medical problem.

## The History

Ask about:

1. Symptoms, e.g., cough and sputum, dyspnoea, wheeze, impaired exercise tolerance, ankle oedema.
2. Precipitating causes of disease exacerbation, e.g., an upper respiratory tract infection, pneumonia, omission of drugs, heart failure, resumption of smoking, pneumothorax.
3. Smoking habit. Ask about number of cigarettes per day and length of use. Ten years of heavy smoking is usually a prerequisite. Absence of a smoking history weighs heavily against the diagnosis unless chronic asthma or alpha-1 antitrypsin deficiency is present.
4. Occupational history. This may be important, particularly as an additive feature if the patient has pneumoconiosis.
5. Medications, especially steroids.
6. Management at home and work.
7. Family history, e.g., alpha-1 antitrypsin deficiency causing emphysema (autosomal recessive: responsible for 2% of cases overall).

## The Examination (p. 160)

Examine the respiratory system carefully. Look particularly for:

1. Pursed lip breathing and use of accessory muscles.
2. Cyanosis and polycythaemia (N.B. clubbing does not occur unless another disease has supervened, e.g., carcinoma).
3. Intercostal recession.
4. Prolonged forced expiratory time.
5. Tracheal tug.
6. Reduced diaphragmatic movements. Overinflation. Reduced chest wall movement and expansion.
7. Reduced breath sounds with or without wheeze (rhonchi).
8. Sputum.
9. Signs of right heart failure.

## Investigations

1. Chest X-ray film—look for signs of emphysema and cor pulmonale.
2. Ventilatory function tests—look for a considerable reduction of the $FEV_1/FVC$ ratio. Vital capacity or total lung capacity may be falsely decreased if measured by gas dilution techniques due to the inhomogeneity of ventilation in chronic obstructive pulmonary disease.
3. Arterial blood gas levels—look for respiratory failure (p. 50).
4. The haemoglobin value—look for polycythaemia (p. 82).
5. Sputum culture which will usually grow *Haemophilus influenzae* or *Streptococcus pneumoniae*.
6. Electrocardiogram—look for signs of right ventricular hypertrophy.

## Differential Diagnosis

1. Asthma.
2. Bronchiectasis.

Features suggesting asthma:

1. Non-smoking patient;
2. Onset in childhood;
3. Family history of allergy;
4. Episodic attacks and also nocturnal symptoms;
5. A rapid response to treatment, especially steroids;
6. Eosinophilia in the sputum.

Features suggesting bronchiectasis:

1. Daily sputum production with or without haemoptysis;
2. Onset in childhood;
3. Recurrent chest infection;
4. Clubbing.

## Treatment

1. Stop smoking. This decreases sputum production and bronchospasm, and may reduce the rate of decline in lung function.
2. Antibiotics to shorten exacerbations (long-term chemoprophylaxis is not generally useful), e.g., amoxycillin given as a course at home at the first sign of purulent sputum.
3. Regular bronchodilators. Beta-2 agonists form the basis of treatment. A home nebulizer may be useful. A small change in $FEV_1$ and FVC may produce considerable subjective improvement. Oral theophylline derivatives may have an additive effect with beta agonists, perhaps because they improve respiratory muscle function. Ipratropium may be of benefit even if the patient has not responded to beta agonists. Inhaled steroids are probably not helpful.

4. Chest physiotherapy and assisted coughing for sputum retention. Maintain adequate hydration.
5. Steroids. Steroid use may be effective in an acute exacerbation. A trial of high doses for 2 weeks may be beneficial when bronchodilators are insufficient. Maintenance steroid treatment should be given only if a short course has been shown objectively to be effective (i.e., improved respiratory function test results). Use the lowest dose possible.
6. Influenza vaccine and pneumococcal vaccine.
7. Exercise and weight reduction increases the patient's well-being, but not lung function.
8. Domiciliary oxygen. This is indicated for patients with a $PaO_2$ of less than 7.33kPa (55mmHg), or cor pulmonale and a $PaO_2$ of less than 7.86kPa (59mmHg). There is evidence that mortality rates are decreased by the use of domiciliary low-flow oxygen given for 16 hours per day.
9. Treatment of cor pulmonale. Treat heart failure together with the lung disease. Avoid digoxin and watch for hypokalaemia.
10. Alpha-1 antitrypsin deficiency can be treated by replenishing the missing antiprotease, which re-establishes antineutrophil elastase protection for the lower lung zones. An intravenous preparation can be administered weekly or monthly.

# PULMONARY FIBROSIS

Infiltrative lung disease has a prolonged course, so patients are often available for the examinations. Discovering the aetiology may be a difficult problem.

## The History

The diagnosis may not be obvious until you examine the patient, at which stage you may have to return and ask further questions.

1. Presenting respiratory symptoms, e.g., dry cough, dyspnoea.
2. Does the patient know the cause of the respiratory symptoms?
3. Systemic symptoms, e.g., weight loss, fatigue, fever, rash, and arthralgia which may indicate a systemic disease, particularly a connective tissue disease or sarcoidosis (Table 6-7).
4. Drug use, e.g., hydralazine, busulphan, nitrofurantoin, bleomycin, cyclophosphamide, methotrexate, procainamide, d-penicillamine, amiodarone.
5. A detailed occupational history, e.g., mineral dust (silicosis, asbestosis, coal miner's pneumoconiosis), chemical fumes (nitrogen dioxide, chlorine, ammonia), organic dusts (Table 6-8).
6. Any history of radiotherapy.
7. History of extrinsic allergic alveolitis (e.g., bird fancier's lung, humidifier lung, farmer's lung, etc.).
8. Infections, e.g., miliary tuberculosis or influenza.
9. Investigations, e.g., lung biopsy or bronchial lavage.

**Table 6-7.** *Fibrotic and Granulomatous Lung Disease*

| | |
|---|---|
| **Connective Tissue Diseases Causing Fibrosis:** | Sarcoidos |
| 1. Rheumatoid Arthritis (p. 92) | P neumocaniosis |
| 2. Systemic Lupus Erythematosus (p. 97) | Ext allergic alveoliks |
| 3. Scleroderma (p. 102) | Connective tissue |
| 4. Polymyositis and Dermatomyositis | Tuberculosis |
| 5. Sjögren's Syndrome (p. 93) | |
| 6. Polyarteritis nodosa (rare) | Rx - Prescribed drugs |
| **Causes of Granulomatous Lung Disease on Lung Biopsy:** | Unknown/ Idiopathic |
| 1. Sarcoidosis (p. 58) | |
| 2. Tuberculosis | Misc - Lymphangioleiomyomatosis |
| 3. Chronic Berylliosis | Histiocytosis X |
| 4. Extrinsic Allergic Alveolitis | Neurofibromatosis |
| | Uraemia  Radiation |

**Table 6-8.** *Asbestos and the Lung*

*Heavy exposure associated with:*
1. Asbestosis
2. Bronchial carcinoma

*Trivial exposure associated with:*
1. Pleural fibrosis and plaques
2. Mesothelioma after a latent period of 30 to 40 years

10. Treatment, if any.
11. Social problems due to the chronic disability.

# The Examination (p. 160)

Clubbing, cyanosis, and crackles (fine, late, inspiratory) make the diagnosis likely. Look for signs of sarcoidosis and connective tissue disease.

# Investigations

Chest radiography is the initial investigation (pp. 171–2). Note whether there is a localized or diffuse abnormality or progressive massive fibrosis (caused by silicosis and coal miner's lung). Pulmonary function tests will reveal a restrictive pattern with reduction of lung volumes, and reduced transfer factor. Blood gas levels will show hypoxia with a normal or low arterial $PaCO_2$. The ESR is often raised. Eosinophilia may be a useful clue (Table 6-9). Serological testing for connective tissue diseases is helpful. Broncheoalveolar lavage and transbronchial lung biopsy are frequently performed—it is suggested that fibrosis associated with a lavage showing a predominance of polymorphonuclear cells is less responsive to treatment. A positive Gallium-67 lung scan may also indicate disease activity. Diagnoses likely to be made by transbronchial lung biopsy include sarcoidosis and lymphangitic spread of carcinoma. Open lung biopsy may be required to confirm idiopathic pulmonary fibrosis.

**Table 6-9.** *Causes of Pulmonary Infiltrate and Peripheral Eosinophilia (PIE)*

**Mnemonic PLATE:**

P.  Prolonged pulmonary eosinophilia—this may be due to: (i) drugs (e.g., sulphonamides, sulphasalazine, salicylates, nitrofurantoin, penicillin, isoniazid, methotrexate, carbamazepine, imipramine, L-tryptophan); (ii) parasites (e.g., ascaris); (iii) idiopathic
L.  Loeffler's syndrome (benign and acute)
A.  Allergic bronchopulmonary aspergillosis (always associated with asthma)
T.  Tropical, e.g., microfilaria
E.  Eosinophilic pneumonia and vasculitis (e.g., polyarteritis nodosa, Wegener's granulomatosis)

**Table 6-10.** *Causes of Pulmonary Fibrosis*

**Upper Lobe (SCHAT):**
S   Silicosis (progressive massive fibrosis); sarcoidosis
C   Coal workers' pneumoconiosis (progressive massive fibrosis)
H   Histiocytosis X
A   Ankylosing spondylitis; allergic bronchopulmonary aspergillosis, allergic alveolitis (may affect the upper or lower lobes)
T   Tuberculosis

**Lower Lobe (RASIO):**
R   Rheumatoid arthritis (p. 92)
A   Asbestosis
S   Scleroderma
I    Idiopathic pulmonary fibrosis, i.e., diffuse fibrosing alveolitis
O   Other, e.g., radiation, drugs (e.g., busulphan, bleomycin, nitrofurantoin, hydralazine, methotrexate, amiodarone)

## Treatment

This depends on the cause (Table 6-10). Remove exposure if appropriate. Steroids may help in diffuse fibrosing alveolitis, chemical injuries, hypersensitivity pneumonias, sarcoidosis, histiocytosis X, and connective tissue disease. They are of no value in dust diseases. A trial of high doses of prednisolone for six weeks may be worthwhile, but follow-up with measurement of spirometry, lung volumes, and transfer factor is important to document response to treatment. Immunosuppressive agents are of unproven benefit, except for their steroid-sparing action. Unilateral lung transplantation may be considered for some patients in the final stage of their disease.

# SARCOIDOSIS

This chronic granulomatous disease is relatively common; patients may require admission to hospital for investigation or treatment and thus be available for the candidate to examine. The prevalence is between 10 and 40 per 100 000 population. Although most patients present between the ages of 20 and 40 years, children and elderly people may sometimes be affected.

## The History

1. Ask why the patient is in hospital. He or she may already know the diagnosis and be in hospital for further investigations or treatment, or the diagnosis may be suspected because of lymphadenopathy or changes on chest X-ray (most patients present with asymptomatic hilar adenopathy).
2. Ask about acute or subacute symptoms, since sarcoidosis develops in this way in about one-third of cases. The patient may have fever, weight loss, loss of appetite and malaise. The occurrence of erythema nodosum, joint symptoms, and bilateral hilar adenopathy on chest X-ray suggests an acute presentation.
3. Symptoms suggesting a more insidious onset include persistent cough and dyspnoea. If the patient has chronic sarcoidosis it is still important to find out how he or she originally presented since the insidious onset is more often associated with chronic sarcoidosis and the development of damage to the lungs and other organs.
4. Ask about skin eruptions, e.g., erythema nodosum, plaques, maculopapular lesions, and subcutaneous nodules.
5. Eye symptoms occur in about one-quarter of patients. The patient may have noticed blurred vision, excess tears and light sensitivity. Involvement of the lacrimal glands can cause the sicca syndrome, resulting in dry, sore eyes.
6. Ask about nasal stuffiness since the nasal mucosa is involved in about one-fifth of patients; occasionally a hoarse voice results from sarcoid involving the larynx.
7. Renal involvement is uncommon but occasionally nephrolithiasis can result because of hypercalcaemia.
8. Ask about neurological symptoms—facial nerve palsy is the most common manifestation, but psychiatric disturbances and fits may occur.
9. Almost half of patients at some time in the course of the disease have arthralgia; even frank arthritis can occur.
10. The patient may be aware of cardiac abnormalities. Conduction problems including complete heart block and ventricular arrhythmias occur in about 5% of patients.
11. If the patient is a woman, ask about pregnancies. Sarcoidosis tends to abate in pregnancy but then flare up postpartum.
12. Inquire about gastrointestinal symptoms, though these are very rare (e.g. dysphagia from hilar adenopathy).
13. Ask how the diagnosis was made. Specifically determine whether a lymph node biopsy or closed or open lung biopsy has been performed. Sometimes a skin or conjunctival biopsy may have been used to make the diagnosis. If the diagnosis was made some time ago, the Kveim reaction may have been tested.

Here an intradermal injection of sarcoid spleen extract is given and then biopsied six weeks later. Typical sarcoid skin lesions develop at the injection site in about 80% of people with sarcoidosis but about 5% of positive results are false-positive tests. Kveim extract is no longer available and bronchial or transbronchial lung biopsies are now used to make the diagnosis in most cases. Occasionally mediastinoscopy with lymph node biopsy is needed to make the diagnosis.

14. Ask about treatment. Find out whether the patient has been receiving steroids and what dose is currently being taken. Various other treatments may have been tried including non-steroidal anti-inflammatory drugs, cyclosporin and cyclophosphamide.

## The Examination (p. 160)

Begin with the examination of the skin. You might be lucky enough to find erythema nodosum. These raised purple lesions are most commonly found on the legs, face and buttocks. Look at the face, back, and extremities for maculopapular eruptions. These are elevated spots less than 1 cm in diameter which have a waxy flat top. There may also be lupus pernio on the face. These are purple swollen nodules with a shiny surface and affect particularly the nose, cheeks, lids, and ears. They may make the nose appear bulbous; occasionally the mucosa of the nose may be involved, and the underlying bone can be destroyed. Lupus pernio may sometimes also involve the fingers and knees. Pink nodules may be found in old scars.

Examine the eyes for signs of uveitis. Yellow conjunctival nodules may be present. Examine the fundi for papilloedema. Uveoparotid fever presents with uveitis, parotid swelling, and VII nerve palsy and fever.

Next examine the respiratory system. Most commonly the physical examination of the chest reveals no abnormality. Look particularly for signs of interstitial lung disease; basal end-inspiratory crackles may be present. Pleural effusions occur rarely.

Next examine all the lymph nodes. Lymphadenopathy may sometimes be generalized. Now examine the abdomen for hepatomegaly (20%) and splenomegaly (up to 40%).

Examine the joints for signs of arthritis which is almost always non-deforming.

Examine the nervous system. Look particularly for facial nerve palsy.

Feel the pulse (heart block or arrhythmia) and look for signs of right ventricular failure or cardiomyopathy.

## Investigations

A full blood count may reveal lymphocytopenia and sometimes eosinophilia. The ESR is often raised. There may be hyperglobulinaemia. The angiotensin-converting enzyme level is raised in about two-thirds of patients with active sarcoidosis but unfortunately is also sometimes elevated in healthy persons or those with primary biliary cirrhosis, leprosy, atypical myobacterial infection, miliary tubercu-

**Table 6-11.** *Chest X-Ray Changes in Sarcoidosis*

1. Hilar lymphadenopathy—up to 90%
2. Paratrachael lymphadenopathy—less than 80%
3. Reticulonodular changes—70%
4. Peripheral nodules—less than 5%
5. Cavitation—less than 5%
6. Pleural effusion—less than 5%
7. Linear atelectasis—less than 1%

losis, silicosis, acute histoplasmosis and hyperparathyroidism. Hypercalcaemia and hypercalciuria may be present.

The chest X-ray is usually abnormal (Table 6-11) and the changes can be classified into 3 stages.

*Stage 1* Bilateral hilar lymphadenopathy.

*Stage 2* Bilateral hilar lymphadenopathy and pulmonary infiltration.

*Stage 3* Pulmonary infiltration without hilar lymphadenopathy.

Patients with stage 1 X-rays are considered to have an acute reversible form of the disease whereas the other stages tend to be more chronic. The chest X-ray may show paratracheal lymphadenopathy; cavitation and pleural effusions are rare. Cavities may become colonized with *Aspergillus*.

Respiratory function tests reveal the changes typical of interstitial lung disease with reduced lung volumes and diffusing capacity but a normal $FEV_1/FVC$ ratio. Occasionally a mixed pattern of obstruction and restriction is seen. Blood gas estimations may show mild hypoxaemia.

A Gallium-67 lung scan usually shows a pattern of diffuse uptake. Enlarged nodes also tend to show up on the scans.

Bronchoscopy with transbronchial biopsy will usually establish the pathological diagnosis. Biopsy of lymph nodes, skin or liver may be diagnostic. The non-caseating granuloma found in sarcoid is non-specific; these are also found in berylliosis, leprosy, hypersensitivity pneumonitis, Crohn's disease, granulomatous infection and in lymph nodes draining adjacent carcinomas.

## Treatment

Most patients recover without treatment. Indications for treatment are lack of resolution of active pulmonary sarcoidosis with impaired lung function, neurological or cardiac complications, major eye disease, and occasionally severe systemic symptoms (e.g., fever, weight loss). Prednisone is the drug of choice if the patient requires therapy.

# CYSTIC FIBROSIS

The survival of children with cystic fibrosis into adult life is now common. Over 50% of patients now reach the age of 20 and prognosis is improving all the time.

Although paediatricians are often reluctant to give these patients up, they are increasingly coming under the care of physicians. They unfortunately tend to spend long periods in hospital and are thus readily available for clinical exams.

Cystic fibrosis is the most common serious congenital inherited defect in Caucasian people. It has an autosomal recessive inheritance, and the gene has been identified. The trait is present in about 1 in 40 Caucasians; 1 in 2000 Caucasians has the condition. It is very rare in other races. It is a chronic disease which can affect the lungs, pancreas, bowel, liver and sweat glands.

## The History

Ask about:

1. Presentation
   (a) The age at diagnosis—milder forms are sometimes not diagnosed until adult life.
   (b) The presenting symptoms—the patient may have been told he or she had meconium ileus as a baby or recurrent respiratory infections in early life. Failure to thrive may have suggested the diagnosis.
   (c) Pulmonary symptoms—cough and sputum, haemoptysis, wheeze, dyspnoea.
   (d) Nasal polyps and sinusitis—relatively common.
   (e) Gastrointestinal symptoms—problems maintaining weight, constipation.
   (f) Heat exhaustion in hot weather. Patients with cystic fibrosis can lose large amounts of salt in their sweat. This can sometimes cause problems, particularly in the tropics.
   (g) Cardiac symptoms—the patient may know of cardiac involvement (cor pulmonale is a late development).
   (h) Jaundice—focal biliary cirrhosis occurs occasionally.
   (i) Diabetes mellitus occurs in 10% of patients with cystic fibrosis.
2. Diagnosis
   The patient may know whether a sweat test was performed. Collection of sweat and measurement of the chloride concentration is still the accepted method of diagnosing the condition. Otherwise a combination of respiratory and malabsorptive problems may be considered enough to make the diagnosis. A list of the major and minor diagnostic criteria is presented in Table 6-12.
3. Family History
   The autosomal recessive inheritance means siblings and other close relatives may well be affected.
4. Treatment
   Pulmonary disease is the main determinant of mortality. Aggressive treatment of the pulmonary complications has had the greatest effect on improvement in life expectancy. The patients are usually well aware of this and are largely responsible for their own treatment. The condition is a chronic suppurative progressive one causing bronchiolitis, bronchitis, pneumonia, and eventually bronchiectasis. The pathology is probably the result of the formation of viscous mucous plugs, which lead to distal infection and lung damage. The mainstay of

treatment is physiotherapy which the patient, with help from the family and a physiotherapist, will perform. Ask about deep breathing, percussion, postural drainage, and the forced expiratory technique 'huffing'. Mucolytic drugs are of very doubtful benefit and may even be harmful. The patient should also know what antibiotics have been used and whether continuously or intermittently. Nebulized bronchodilators and antibiotics are commonly prescribed. Ask whether treatment for complications like pneumothorax, haemoptysis or cor pulmonale has been required. Minor haemoptysis where less than 250mL of blood is lost occurs in about 60% of patients. Major haemoptysis occurs in about 7% and bronchial artery embolization may be required. Cor pulmonale may require treatment with diuretics. Pleurodesis used to be the treatment of choice for recurrent pneumothorax, but it is probably an absolute contraindication to heart-lung transplant.

5. Gastrointestinal
   This tends to be less of a problem, but malabsorption may make weight gain very difficult for these patients. Ask what pancreatic enzyme replacement the patient uses and how often.

6. Ask about the number of admissions to hospital over the last 12 months and the length of each stay. There is some evidence that routine admission to hospital 3 or 4 times a year for intensive physiotherapy and nebulized antibiotics and bronchodilators may be beneficial.

7. Social Support
   Ask whether the patient knows about or belongs to the local Cystic Fibrosis Association and whether he or she has been in touch with other affected patients. Try to find out tactfully whether the patient understands the inheritance of the disease; male patients may know that azoospermia is usually present (95%).

## The Examination (p. 160)

Look at the patient's size and physique. Muscle bulk is considered a good indicator of the severity and prognosis in a particular patient. Measure or estimate the patient's stature and weight.

Ask the patient to cough. Listen for a loose cough and examine any sputum for the degree of purulence. Now examine the respiratory system carefully. Note clubbing which is present in the majority of patients. Look for abnormal chest wall development. Estimate forced expiratory time and examine the chest listening particularly for crackles, wheezes and reduced breath sounds.

Examine the heart for signs of cor pulmonale and right ventricular failure.

## Investigations

Sputum culture is most important. Colonization with *Haemophilus influenzae* tends to occur in young patients, and this is often followed by nosocomial *Escherichia coli* and *Proteus* spp. Older patients tend to have *Staphylococcus aureus*. By the age of 10 years, pseudomonas is the main pathogen in most patients, but usually

**Table 6-12.** *Diagnosis of Cystic Fibrosis*

**Major Criteria**
1. Elevated chloride sweat test (98%)—pilocarpine iontophoresis on 100mg of sweat
   >70mmol/L—diagnostic in adults
   >60mmol/L—diagnostic in children
   50 to 60mmol/L—suggestive
   <50mmol/L—normal
2. Azoospermia in males (95%)
3. Family history of cystic fibrosis (70%)

**Minor Criteria**
1. Nasal polyps (relatively uncommon)
2. Meconium ileus equivalent (distal bowel obstruction from inspissated secretions)
3. Rectal prolapse
4. Focal biliary cirrhosis
5. Diabetes mellitus (uncommon)

it does not cause systemic infection. Pseudomonas is resistant to many antibiotics, although ciprofloxacin is often effective when taken orally and there is some evidence that the long-term use of this drug is effective. Otherwise a nebulized aminoglycoside should probably be used regularly.

A blood count to look for anaemia which may be due to malabsorption or chronic disease should be asked for; the white cell count may indicate acute infection. The electrolyte levels liver function tests and blood sugar levels should be looked at. The creatinine level should be known before aminoglycosides are used. The chest X-ray should be looked at carefully and should be compared with previous films if these are available. Increased lung markings are present in 98% of patients. These occur particularly in the upper lobes. Cystic bronchiectatic changes occur in over 60% of patients. Mucous plugs may be seen in a third and atelectasis occurs in just over 10% of patients. Look also for pneumothorax and pleural changes at the site of previous pneumothoraces or pleurodesis.

## Management

Intensive and repetitive physiotherapy is the mainstay of treatment. You should try to form an idea of the patient's ability to cope with the illness since so much of the management depends on him or her. Malabsorption may require aggressive treatment with pancreatic enzyme supplements and frequent small meals as well as vitamin supplements. Combined heart and lung transplantation is now an accepted, although still uncommon, treatment in patients with advanced disease. Cystic fibrosis does not recur in the transplanted lung.

# MALABSORPTION

This is a difficult long case. It is usually a diagnostic problem.

## The History

Ask about:

1. Presenting symptoms, e.g.:
   (a) pale, bulky, offensive stools (steatorrhoea);
   (b) weight loss;
   (c) weakness (potassium deficiency);
   (d) anaemia (megaloblastic, iron-deficiency, etc.)
   (e) bone pain (osteomalacia);
   (f) glossitis and angular stomatitis (vitamin B group deficiency);
   (g) bruising (vitamin K deficiency);
   (h) oedema due to protein deficiency;
   (i) peripheral neuropathy due to $B_{12}$ or $B_1$ deficiency;
   (j) skin rash (eczema, dermatitis herpetiformis);
   (k) amenorrhoea due to protein depletion.
2. Time of onset of symptoms and their duration.
3. Aetiological questions:
   (a) gastrectomy, other bowel surgery;
   (b) history of liver or pancreatic disease;
   (c) drugs, e.g., alcohol, neomycin, cholestyramine;
   (d) history of Crohn's disease;
   (e) previous radiotherapy;
   (f) gluten-free diet treatment at any stage;
   (g) history of diabetes mellitus.
4. Current treatment, e.g., diet, pancreatic supplements, vitamin supplements, cholestyramine, antibiotics.
5. Family history, e.g., coeliac disease, inflammatory bowel disease.
6. Social problems related to the chronic illness.

## The Examination (p. 165)

Pay particular attention in the gastrointestinal system to abdominal scars, nutritional state, skin lesions (e.g., bruising, dermatitis herpetiformis, erythema nodosum, pyoderma gangrenosum, stomatitis, pigmentation, perianal lesions), signs of anaemia, signs of chronic liver disease, peripheral neuropathy and lymphadenopathy.

## Investigations (Table 6-13)

1. Demonstrate malabsorption:
   (a) faecal fat estimation over 3 days—greater than 7g per day is abnormal;
   (b) Schilling test for ileal disease;
   (c) xylose test for jejunal disease (of minor value).
2. Evaluate the consequences:
   (a) blood count with particular attention to red cell indices;
   (b) serum iron and ferritin, serum and red cell folate, and $B_{12}$ studies;
   (c) serum albumin estimation;

**Table 6-13.**  *Typical Results of Investigations in Malabsorption*

| Investigation | Coeliac Disease | Bacterial Overgrowth | Whipple's Disease | Terminal Ileal Disease | Chronic Pancreatitis |
|---|---|---|---|---|---|
| Stool fat (or C14 triolein breath test) | High | High | High | High | Very high |
| D-Xylose* | Low | Low | Low | Normal | Normal |
| Schilling's test with or without IF† | Normal (rarely abnormal due to ileal involvement) | Abnormal ileal involvement | Normal | Abnormal | Abnormal occasionally |
| Folate (serum) | Low(in >50%) | High to normal | Low | Normal | Normal |
| Small bowel biopsy (proximal) | Subtotal or total villous atrophy | Normal (>10⁵ organisms on quantitative jejunal fluid culture) | Clubbing and flattening of villi, PAS-positive macrophages | Normal | Normal |
| C14 glycocholate breath test | Normal | Abnormal (usually early peak) | Normal | Abnormal (late peak) | Normal |

\*   This is a test of proximal small bowel function. Falsely low values occur in chronic renal failure, dehydration, ascites, hyperthyroidism and in the elderly.

†   While pernicious anemia corrects with intrinsic factor (IF), ileal disease does not correct. Bacterial overgrowth corrects with antibiotics and pancreatic insufficiency with pancreatic supplements. False-negative results occur with incomplete urinary collections, decreased extracellular volume and renal disease.

PAS = periodic acid—Schiff technique.

    (d) vitamin D assay, serum calcium, phosphate and alkaline phosphatase estimations;

    (e) clotting profile—prothrombin index.

3. Find the cause:

    (a) Small bowel X-ray films for localized disease, e.g., Crohn's disease or anatomical causes of bacterial overgrowth such as diverticula or blind loops.

    (b) Small bowel biopsy and duodenal aspirate for histology, parasites and bacterial overgrowth. Subtotal villous atrophy may be present in:

        (i)    coeliac disease;

        (ii)   tropical sprue;

        (iii)  giardiasis;

        (iv)   lymphoma;

        (v)    hypogammaglobulinaemia;

        (vi)   Whipple's disease.

    (c) B₁₂ absorption may be abnormal in ileal disease, bacterial overgrowth, pernicious anaemia and pancreatic disease.

**Table 6-14.** *Causes and Treatment of Malabsorption*

**1. Lipolytic Phase Defects:**
   *Causes*, e.g.:
   a) Chronic pancreatitis
   b) Cystic fibrosis
   *Treatment*:
   a) Reverse causes
   b) Pancreatic enzyme supplements
   c) Medium chain triglycerides

**2. Micellar Phase Defects:**
   *Causes*, e.g.:
   a) Extrahepatic biliary obstruction
   b) Chronic liver disease (p. 72)
   c) Bacterial overgrowth
   d) Terminal ileal disease [e.g., Crohn's disease (p. 68)] or resection
   *Treatment*:
   a) Reverse causes (e.g., antibiotics for bacterial overgrowth)
   b) Cholestyramine if bile acid cathartic effect is important (e.g., less than 100cm ileum resected and no steatorrhoea)
   c) Medium chain triglycerides for steatorrhoea (e.g., more than 100cm ileum resected)
   d) Fat-soluble vitamin supplements

**3. Mucosal and Delivery Phase Defects:**
   *Causes*, e.g.:
   a) Coeliac disease (Table 6-15)
   b) Tropical sprue
   c) Lymphoma (p. 87), intestinal lymphangiectasia
   d) Whipple's disease
   e) Small bowel ischaemia, resection
   f) Amyloidosis
   g) Hypogammaglobulinaemia
   h) HIV infection (Kaposi's sarcoma, idiopathic)
   *Treatment*:
   a) Reverse causes, e.g., gluten-free diet (coeliac disease), antibiotics (Whipple's disease)
   b) Fat-soluble vitamin supplements

(d) The bile acid (C14 glycocholate) breath test is used to detect bacterial overgrowth and ileal disease. The C14 xylose test is more sensitive and specific for the detection of bacterial overgrowth.

(e) Greatly raised faecal fat levels (over 40g per day) strongly suggests pancreatic disease. This is investigated by plain abdominal X-ray films (for calcification), abdominal ultrasound and/or CT scan, and endoscopic retrograde cholangiopancreatography (ERCP). Pancreatic function testing may be useful in selected cases.

## Treatment

Treatment depends on the cause and also involves the replacement of essential nutrients (Table 6-14).

**Table 6-15.** *Coeliac Disease*

**Diagnostic Criteria for Coeliac Disease:**
1. Evidence of malabsorption
2. Abnormal jejunal biopsy
3. Clinical, biochemical and histological improvement on a gluten-free diet (no wheat, rye or barley)
4. Relapse on reinstitution of gluten (not recommended in adults)
      N.B.  Splenomegaly in coeliac disease usually indicates that lymphoma has complicated the disease, because otherwise splenic atrophy is characteristic and manifests with Howell-Jolly bodies in the peripheral blood smear.

**Causes of Lack of Response to a Gluten-Free Diet:**
1. Incorrect diagnosis
2. Patient not adhering to the diet
3. Collagenous sprue
4. Intestinal lymphoma
5. Diffuse ulceration
6. Other intercurrent disease

**Complications of Coeliac Disease:**
1. T-cell lymphoma (p. 87)
2. Ulceration of the small bowel
3. Carcinoma of the gastrointestinal tract is generally slightly increased

Coeliac disease (Table 6-15), chronic pancreatitis and previous gastric surgery account for 60% of cases of malabsorption.

# INFLAMMATORY BOWEL DISEASE

Both ulcerative colitis and Crohn's disease are common conditions in hospitals. They present both diagnostic and management problems. For these reasons, this type of long case is very common. The patient will usually know the diagnosis, but you may have to decide which type of inflammatory bowel disease is present.

## The History

Ask about:

1. Symptoms at presentation and current reason for admission. Ulcerative colitis typically presents in young adults with relapsing bloody diarrhoea, malaise, fever and weight loss. Crohn's disease has a variable presentation, including an insidious onset of pain, diarrhoea, weight loss, malabsorption, intestinal obstruction, and 'appendicitis'.
2. Local complications of the disease (Table 6-16).
3. Extracolonic manifestations of the disease (Table 6-16).
4. Sexual preference (infective proctitis in homosexuals must be considered).
5. Investigations at the time of presentation and subsequently (and particularly whether infectious causes were considered).

**Table 6-16.** *Complications of Inflammatory Bowel Disease*

**Ulcerative Colitis**

*Local:*
1. Toxic megacolon (diameter of colon more than 6cm, on plain abdominal X-ray film)
2. Perforation
3. Massive haemorrhage
4. Strictures
5. Carcinoma of the colon—often multicentric and related to disease extent and duration

*Extracolonic:*
1. Liver disease:
   a) fatty liver
   b) sclerosing cholangitis (large duct or small duct [pericholangitis])
   c) chronic active hepatitis
   d) cirrhosis
   e) carcinoma of the bile duct
   f) amyloidosis (very rare)
2. Blood disorders:
   a) anaemia (due to chronic disease, iron deficiency, ileal involvement, haemolysis from sulphasalazine or microangiopathy)
   b) thromboembolism (due to antithrombin III deficiency, stasis, dehydration)
3. Arthropathy:
   a) peripheral (large joints)
   b) ankylosing spondylitis (p. 204)
4. Skin and mucous membranes:
   a) erythema nodosum (coincides with active disease) (p. 60)
   b) pyoderma gangrenosum
   c) aphthous ulcers
5. Ocular—uveitis, conjunctivitis, episcleritis

**Crohn's Disease**

*Local:*
1. Anorectal disease (including anal fissures or fistulas, pararectal abscess or rectovaginal fistula)
2. Obstruction (usually terminal ileum)
3. Fistula
4. Toxic megacolon and perforation (rare)
5. Carcinoma of the small and large bowel (increased only slightly)

*Extracolonic:*
Similar to ulcerative colitis except for the following:
1. Liver disease—sclerosing cholangitis is less common
2. Gallstones are increased (due to decreased bile salt pool)
3. Renal complications include urate and calcium oxalate stones, pyelonephritis (due to fistulas), hydronephrosis (ureteric obstruction), amyloidosis
4. Malabsorption due to small bowel involvement
5. Osteomalacia

**Table 6-17.**  *Causes of Colitis*

1. Inflammatory bowel disease
2. Infections including pseudomembranous colitis
3. Radiation
4. Ischaemic colitis or ischaemia associated with the oral contraceptive pill
5. Diversion colitis (in colon loops excluded from the faecal stream)
6. Toxic exposure, e.g., peroxide or soapsud enemas, gold-induced colitis

6. The number of hospital admissions.
7. Whether regular follow-up colonoscopy has been performed in patients with ulcerative colitis.
8. Treatment—medications, e.g., sulphasalazine, local or systemic steroids, metronidazole, other antibiotics, surgery.
9. Family history of inflammatory bowel disease or of bowel carcinoma.
10. Domestic arrangements and employment.

## The Examination (p. 165)

A thorough gastrointestinal system examination is important. Evaluate the general state of nutrition and hydration. Feel for any tenderness or abdominal masses and look for anal lesions externally. Always ask for the results of a rectal examination and urine analysis. Look for the signs of Cushing's syndrome if the patient is taking steroids. Search for the other extracolonic manifestations, being guided by the history, e.g., arthropathy, skin lesions, uveitis, anaemia, liver disease, etc.

## Investigations

It is important to exclude other causes of colitis (Table 6-17). For the investigation of inflammatory bowel disease the following should be considered:

1. Infection must be excluded. The causes include amoebiasis (diagnosed by rectal mucosal scraping or warm stool examination), *Shigella, Salmonella, Yersinia, Campylobacter, E. coli* 0157:H7 and pseudomembranous colitis (*Clostridium difficile*). Lymphogranuloma venereum (a chlamydial disease which is sexually transmitted), gonorrhoea and syphilis (particularly in homosexuals) and other infections in immunocompromised hosts (e.g., herpes, cytomegalovirus, cryptosporidium, *Isospora belli*) should be considered in patients at risk.
2. Sigmoidoscopy and biopsy. Inspect for decreased mucosal translucency, loss of vascular pattern, granular and friable mucosa, hyperaemia, ulceration and pseudopolyps.
3. Plain abdominal X-ray film. It is important to look for bowel wall thickening (oedema), gaseous distension and evidence of toxic megacolon in ulcerative colitis. In Crohn's disease also look for loops of matted bowel and small bowel obstruction.

4. Blood count. Check for anaemia (due to chronic disease, blood loss, macrocytic anaemia in ileal disease, or haemolytic anaemia from an autoimmune process, microangiopathic disease or sulphasalazine).
5. Liver function tests and electrolytes, urea, and creatinine. These patients may develop liver disease as well as renal stones, pyelonephritis, hydronephrosis or amyloidosis. Remember hypoalbuminaemia is a sign of severe disease.
6. Barium enema. This is contraindicated in very active colitis and with toxic megacolon, because of the risk of perforation. This investigation will help distinguish ulcerative colitis from Crohn's disease—in ulcerative colitis the rectum is nearly always involved and there are no skip lesions. Look for loss of haustrations, mucosal irregularity and ulceration, spasm, pseudopolyps and bowel shortening. Also look for evidence of strictures and carcinoma. In Crohn's colitis, look for thickening, 'cobblestoning', luminal narrowing, skip lesions, fistulas, and transverse fissures (sinus tracts).
7. Colonoscopy is a very useful investigation to assess whether disease is patchy or not and its extent. Mucosal biopsies may often not differentiate ulcerative colitis from Crohn's disease. Mucus depletion and prominent crypt abscess formation are more suggestive of ulcerative colitis. Granuloma (in 25%) or focal inflammation is found in Crohn's colitis (but note granulomas also occur in biopsies from homosexual men with *Chlamydia trachomatis*, syphilitic proctitis, or in tuberculosis). Patients with ulcerative colitis who have had pancolitis for more than 7 years or left-sided colitis for 13 years or more should have colonoscopic screening with biopsy every 1 to 3 years to look for high-grade dysplasia and carcinoma. If high-grade dysplasia is confirmed in the absence of severe inflammation, colectomy is indicated. If severe inflammation is present, assessment for dysplasia is necessary after inducing remission of the active inflammation.

## Treatment

### *Ulcerative Colitis*

In ulcerative colitis, grade the severity of the disease:

1. mild—fewer than four motions per day, minimal bleeding;
2. moderate—four to six motions per day, bleeding;
3. severe—more than six motions per day, profuse bleeding.

Other useful indices of severity are fever, tachycardia, anaemia, hypoalbuminaemia and acute phase reactants (e.g., ESR, C-reactive protein).

In an acute attack, remember to correct hypokalaemia and avoid barium enemas to prevent toxic megacolon. Do not prescribe opiates or anticholinergic agents for a similar reason. In severe colitis, intravenous broad spectrum antibiotics (including metronidazole) and hyperalimentation may be given. Steroids are the mainstay of treatment in moderate to severe disease. In mild to moderate disease, sulphasalazine is useful; 5-amino salicylic acid is the active agent, while sulphapyridine is the cause of most intolerance (allergic reactions, e.g., skin rash—

including Stevens-Johnson syndrome—Heinz body haemolytic anaemia; side effects, e.g., nausea, headache, folate deficiency, reversible male infertility). The minimum dose is 2 to 4g per day. Sulphasalazine decreases the relapse rate and administration should be continued indefinitely. 5-amino salicylic acid formulations are also effective for mild to moderate inflammation but have fewer side effects. Chronic steroid use does NOT reduce relapse rates. Close cooperation with a surgeon interested in this field is important in severe disease.

It is important to try to differentiate ulcerative colitis from Crohn's disease based on clinical presentation, X-ray, endoscopic and histologic findings. This is because ulcerative colitis that does not respond to medical management can be cured by colectomy and because patients with extensive ulcerative colitis are at an increased risk of developing colorectal cancer. In 5% to 10% of patients, a specific distinction cannot be made.

Colectomy in ulcerative colitis is curative. Indications for surgery include chronic ill health and severe disease, complications (e.g., perforation, massive bleeding), and severe disease not responding to optimal medical treatment in 10–14 days. Patients with a very high risk of carcinoma (confirmed high-grade dysplasia on biopsy or dysplasia in a lesion or mass) should be advised to undergo a colectomy. All manifestations of the disease are cured by colectomy, but ankylosing spondylitis, liver disease, and occasionally pyoderma gangrenosum do *not* respond. While the standard Brooke ileostomy is the simplest procedure, the ileal pouch anal anastamosis is increasingly being used as it maintains intestinal continuity, although it does leave the patient with 4 to 8 bowel movements daily and may be complicated by pouchitis. The latter usually responds to metronidazole treatment.

### Crohn's Disease

For active disease, treatment is similar to ulcerative colitis. Sulphasalazine is more effective in colonic disease, while steroids are more effective in small bowel disease. In quiescent disease no agent is effective in preventing relapse. Metronidazole is particularly useful for severe perianal disease and fistulae; 6-mercaptopurine may be tried in difficult severe cases. Surgery is reserved for the complications of Crohn's disease (e.g., internal fistula with abscess, intestinal obstruction that does not respond to medical management). The best operation is resection. Strictureplasty may allow relief of localized obstruction without the deleterious effects of multiple resections. When a total colectomy is needed, the standard ileostomy is the procedure of choice. The recurrence rate of the disease is unchanged by surgery.

# CHRONIC LIVER DISEASE

Cirrhosis alone or in combination with other disease will often crop up, particularly in repatriation hospitals. (Warning: you may be exposed to prolonged war stories and discussions about shrapnel.) It is a pathological diagnosis. This discussion will be limited to aspects of cirrhosis and chronic active hepatitis which tend to come up in the examination.

## The History

Cirrhosis presents in three-quarters of cases with jaundice or ascites and in one-quarter with abdominal pain, acute bleeding or encephalopathy. Only occasionally will patients present with just weakness, lassitude or loss of libido. Ask about:

1. Reason for current hospital admission.
2. Length of history of liver disease:
   (a) past history of hepatitis or jaundice including contacts;
   (b) alcohol intake (in men 80g per day for more than 10 years is usually necessary, but women need less exposure);
   (c) history of drug addiction (intravenous), sexual preference, transfusions, etc.
   (d) drug history (e.g., for chronic active hepatitis: methyldopa, isoniazid, nitrofurantoin);
   (e) history of diabetes mellitus, cardiac failure, or arthropathy (haemochromatosis);
   (f) overseas travel (e.g., acute hepatitis)
3. Treatment, e.g., protein restriction, fluid restriction, alcohol abstinence, steroids, lactulose, neomycin.
4. Complications, e.g., any history of encephalopathy, any history of portal hypertension (ascites or bleeding from varices), recent abdominal pain (gallstones—usually pigment stones, acute alcoholic hepatitis, etc.).
5. Investigations, e.g., liver biopsy.
6. Operations, e.g., portacaval shunt.
7. Impotence, loss of libido.
8. Social problems, e.g., employment, family, etc.

## The Examination (p. 165)

*chronic liver disease*
*portal hypertension*
*encephalopathy*

Examine carefully for the signs of chronic liver disease. Also note any hepatic encephalopathy, signs of portal hypertension (splenomegaly, ascites, oedema, caput medusae) and signs of bleeding (e.g., melaena).

Consider hepatocellular carcinoma (particularly in haemochromatosis and cirrhosis due to hepatitis B or C infection). In patients with decompensated cirrhosis, examine for a hard mass and liver bruit (hepatoma). Look for the signs of haemochromatosis (p. 77). In young patients consider Wilson's disease and look carefully for Kayser-Fleischer rings. If there is deep jaundice with scratch marks and xanthelasma, particularly in a woman, consider end-stage primary biliary cirrhosis. Exclude severe right heart failure or constrictive pericarditis clinically in all patients. Other causes and sequelae are given in Tables 6-18 and 6-19.

## Investigations

Management of chronic liver disease depends upon aetiology, morphology and hepatic function. It is important to make a diagnosis and exclude potentially reversible causes of further liver deterioration.

**Table 6-18.** *Causes of Cirrhosis in Adults*

1. Alcohol
2. Postviral (B; C)
3. Cryptogenic (idiopathic)
4. Drugs, e.g. methyldopa, chlorpromazine, isoniazid, nitrofurantoin, propylthiouracil, methotrexate, amiodarone
5. Autoimmune chronic active hepatitis
6. Inflammatory bowel disease    UC
7. Haemochromatosis
8. Wilson's disease
9. Primary biliary cirrhosis
10. Secondary biliary cirrhosis
11. Alpha-1 antitrypsin deficiency
12. Cystic fibrosis
13. Budd-Chiari syndrome, cardiac failure, chronic constrictive pericarditis

**Table 6-19.** *Sequelae of Cirrhosis*

1. Portal hypertension and ascites
2. Portal vein thrombosis (rare)
3. Spontaneous bacterial peritonitis
4. Hepatic encephalopathy
5. Hepatorenal syndrome
6. Hepatocellular carcinoma

*Alb*
*AST ALT*
*YGT Alk phos*

*FBC*
*Coag*

*U+E*

1. Liver function tests. These should be used to confirm abnormalities, follow progress and give an idea of prognosis (particularly albumin level and prothrombin index).
2. Full blood count. This is helpful as anaemia may be due to chronic disease, blood loss, folate deficiency, bone marrow depression, hypersplenism, haemolysis or sideroblastic anaemia. Round macrocytes are common in alcoholics. Remember leucopenia and thrombocytopenia occur in hypersplenism.
3. Renal function tests are important to exclude hepatorenal syndrome.
4. Ascitic tap (Tables 6-20 and 6-21).
5. Ultrasound. This may help exclude biliary obstruction and infiltration. The texture of the liver may suggest nodularity or cirrhotic change.
6. Liver biopsy. This is a definitive test and probably should be done if the diagnosis is uncertain unless there are specific contraindications, e.g., coagulopathy.

Always assess for causative factors (Table 6-18). Hepatitis B and C serology should be obtained. The test for antimitochondrial antibody in primary biliary cirrhosis and those for smooth muscle antibody and antinuclear factor in chronic active hepatitis may be indicated. Iron studies and less commonly caeruloplasmin levels may be ordered. Alpha-1 antitrypsin deficiency should be considered; absence of the alpha-1 fraction on a protein electrophoresis is a useful clue. Evaluate for evidence of inflammatory bowel disease.

**Table 6-20.** *Causes of Ascites and Interpretation of Ascitic Fluid Studies*

*[handwritten: Transudate < 30 Failure]*

**Causes**
1. Transudate (<30g protein/L)
   a) Cirrhosis (and portal hypertension—usually late)
   b) Congestive heart failure, constrictive pericarditis
   c) Hypoalbuminaemia, e.g., nephrotic syndrome (Table 6-35 p. 114)
   d) Meig's syndrome
2. Exudate (>30g protein/L)
   a) Malignant disease (e.g., bowel, gynaecological)
   b) Infection (e.g., tuberculosis, pyogenic)
   c) Pancreatitis
   d) Budd-Chiari syndrome (hepatic vein thrombosis) or inferior vena caval obstruction (Table 6-21)
   e) Lymphatic obstruction (chylous ascites)
   f) Myxoedema

**Examination of Ascitic Fluid Following a Diagnostic Paracentesis**
   a) Protein—distinguishes a transudate from an exudate  *[handwritten: < 30 Transudate]*
   b) Blood—suggests malignancy or a recent invasive test
   c) Turbid or white fluid—suggests infection or chylous ascites
   d) Cell count (0 to 300 mononuclear cells is normal: >500 cells or >250 polymorphs per cubic millimetre suggests spontaneous bacterial peritonitis)
   e) pH <7.35—suggests spontaneous bacterial peritonitis or systemic acidosis
   f) Lactate—increased in spontaneous bacterial peritonitis
   g) Amylase—elevated in pancreatic ascites
   h) Cytology—for malignant cells (false positive results common)
   i) Culture—for spontaneous bacterial peritonitis

Finally, assess the hepatic functional reserve of patients with known or suspected cirrhosis (Table 6-22).

*[handwritten: Alkalosis ⇒ ↑ NH3 across BBB]*
*[handwritten: ↓ K+ ⇒ ↑ Renal NH3 production.]*

## Treatment

This consists of treating hepatocellular failure and portal hypertension. Cirrhosis is irreversible. However, removing causative factors is important, e.g., alcohol, iron overload, drugs.

### Hepatocellular Failure

Acute hepatic encephalopathy is precipitated by bleeding into the gastrointestinal tract or electrolyte disturbances (alkalosis increases the ammonia crossing the blood-brain barrier, while hypokalaemia increases renal ammonia production). Hypokalaemia may be due to recent diuretic use. Infection (e.g., spontaneous bacterial peritonitis), drugs (e.g., sedatives), high protein diet, constipation, deteriorating liver function (e.g., alcoholic binge, hepatoma) and rarely metabolic disturbances (e.g., hypoglycaemia, hypoxia) may also precipitate encephalopathy.

Management consists of removing precipitating factors. This means removing blood from the gut (e.g., enemas), giving a low-protein diet, treating infection,

**Table 6-21.**  *Budd-Chiari Syndrome*

Typically young adults who have pain—due to hepatic congestion—hepatomegaly and ascites.

**Causes**
1. Idiopathic—thrombosis or fibrous obliteration of hepatic vein
2. Myeloproliferative disease, especially polycythaemia rubra vera
3. Malignant disease, e.g., renal, pancreatic, hepatoma, adrenal, testicular, thyroid
4. The contraceptive pill or pregnancy
5. Paroxysmal nocturnal haemoglobinuria (PNH)
6. Drugs, e.g., azathioprine, adriamycin
7. Fibrous membrane, trauma, schistosomiasis, amoebiasis

**Diagnosis**
1. Liver function tests—non-specific, but serum alkaline phosphatase level may be high
2. Ascitic tap (classically an exudate but may be a transudate)
3. Ultrasonography with Doppler flow studies—less sensitive than angiography but diagnostic in >85% of cases
4. Technetium sulphur colloid liver scan (increased caudate lobe uptake)—less useful
5. Liver biopsy (highly suggestive—'nutmeg' liver)
6. Angiography and venography (usually diagnostic)

**Table 6-22.**  *Child's Classification of Patients With Cirrhosis in Terms of Hepatic Functional Reserve*

|  | A | B | C |
|---|---|---|---|
| Degree of impairment | Minimal | Moderate | Severe |
| Serum bilirubin (μmol/L) | <35 | 35 to 50 | >50 |
| Serum albumin (g/L) | >35 | 30 to 35 | <30 |
| (μmol/L) | (>507) | (435–507) | (<435) |
| Ascites | None | Easily controlled | Poorly controlled |
| Encephalopathy | None | Minimal | Advanced; 'coma' |
| Nutrition | Excellent | Good | Poor; 'wasting' |

correcting electrolyte disturbances, avoiding sedatives and attacking the urea-splitting organisms with lactulose or lactilol (lactulose causes more diarrhoea) and/or neomycin.

Chronic hepatocellular failure should be managed by treating the aetiology where possible and manipulating the protein diet as required. Control encephalopathy and ascites. Watch for gastrointestinal bleeding and renal failure. In cases of chronic active hepatitis, steroids may be helpful in patients without viral markers.

## Portal Hypertension

Clinical features include splenomegaly, the presence of collaterals, ascites and fetor hepaticus.

Investigations include endoscopy for oesophageal varices and occasionally measurement of the wedged hepatic venous pressure (WHVP) or portal venography. The WHVP pressure is increased in cirrhosis, but is normal in presinusoidal portal hypertension (e.g., schistosomiasis, portal vein obstruction).

Treatment of ascites consists of gentle diuresis (maximum weight loss of 500g per day). Begin with bed rest and salt restriction. Consider spironolactone 2 to 4 days later, and increase the dose slowly. If the urinary sodium to potassium ratio is greater than 1, a dose of 150mg/day is usually adequate; if the ratio is less than 1, higher doses are needed. Frusemide is given if absolutely necessary. Therapeutic paracentesis is a safe alternative in Child's grade B patients with tense ascites, especially when there is also peripheral oedema. Intravenous salt-poor albumin is given to replace the protein lost in ascitic fluid and 5 to 10L can be removed; the procedure can be repeated if necessary. Therapeutic paracentesis is contraindicated in renal failure or severe coagulopathy. Le Veen shunts are occasionally tried for severe ascites. They do not improve the prognosis. Complications of Le Veen shunting include disseminated intravascular coagulation, infection, cardiac failure, pulmonary oedema and variceal bleeding; shunt failure is common.

Bleeding varices should be managed acutely by replacing blood and correcting coagulation abnormalities. Intravenous vasopressin combined with nitroglycerine is first-line therapy but is only a temporary measure. Oesophageal variceal sclerosis therapy is effective in stopping acute bleeding; oesophageal balloon tamponade is now uncommonly required. To prevent recurrent variceal bleeding, elective endoscopic sclerotherapy to obliterate varices may be effective. Beta-blockers can reduce portal pressure and may be useful in patients with good liver function. Portasystemic shunting is controversial—it probably does not reduce mortality in the long term. Mortality is high for 'crash' shunts.

### Haemochromatosis     A3

This is an autosomal recessive disease. Family members can be tested for the carrier state by determining HLA haplotype. Patients usually present with hepatomegaly and abdominal pain. Hepatoma occurs in 14% of patients with cirrhosis. Diabetes mellitus is common, as is skin pigmentation (from iron and melanin). Dilated cardiomyopathy, arthropathy (p. 182) and testicular atrophy (due to iron deposition in the pituitary gland, not in the testis) also occur.

Diagnosis is suggested by an increased transferrin saturation and a raised ferritin level; liver biopsy to measure iron stores is the definitive test. In difficult cases, phlebotomy will establish how much iron is present.

Iron chelating agents like desferrioxamine are not useful.

Treatment is venesection weekly or as required for approximately 2 years (as 40 to 60g of excess iron is deposited) and then once every 3 months. The avoidance of alcohol is important. Arthropathy and endocrine changes do not respond to treatment. Cirrhosis and diabetes may partially respond. Hepatoma is not prevented by venesection in patients with established cirrhosis.

# LIVER TRANSPLANTATION

Liver transplantation is now an important therapeutic option in the patient with irreversible, progressive liver disease for which there is no acceptable alternative therapy and no absolute contraindication. One-year survival overall is now 75%. In the examination setting a patient will either have chronic liver disease and be a candidate for transplant, or be a transplant recipient who has a problem.

## History

1. Obtain details of the patient's liver disease, including diagnosis and duration. Candidates for liver transplant include patients with cirrhosis (particularly primary biliary or cryptogenic cirrhosis), primary sclerosing cholangitis, autoimmune chronic active hepatitis, chronic portal-systemic encephalopathy, Budd-Chiari syndrome, inherited metabolic diseases (e.g., Wilson's disease, alpha-1 anti-trypsin deficiency) and acute or subacute hepatic failure.
2. If the patient may be a candidate for liver transplant, inquire about potential contraindications. Absolute contraindications include active sepsis outside the liver, metastatic malignancy, cholangiocarcinoma, active alcoholism, AIDS, severe hypoxaemia due to intrapulmonary shunting, diffuse portal vein thrombosis and advanced cardiopulmonary or renal disease. Relative contraindications include advanced age ($\geq$60 years), a prior portacaval shunt, intrahepatic or biliary infection, localized portal vein thrombosis, prior complex hepatobiliary surgery, hepatitis B or HIV infection and renal impairment.
3. Enquire about complications of the patients's liver disease: previous haemorrhages, ascites, pre-coma, etc. The timing of transplant for patients with end-stage chronic disease is important; this should be considered when the patient is invalided but before complications have occurred that preclude proceeding (e.g., preterminal variceal bleeding, irreversible hepatorenal syndrome, development of a catabolic state, irreversible coagulopathy, vascular instability with ascites or incapacitating osteopenic bone disease).
4. If the patient has had a transplant, enquire about the postoperative course, including whether further surgery was carried out (e.g., to drain abscesses; reconstruct the biliary tract; control bleeding; re-transplant for graft failure; hepatic arterial thrombosis). Also inquire about postoperative infections.
5. Ask about complications of liver transplantation. Early on (in the first five days) primary graft failure, technical problems (e.g., bleeding, hepatic arterial thrombosis, bile leaks, portal vein thrombosis), renal failure and pulmonary complications (atelectasis, pleural effusion, infection) may occur. Major problems after discharge from the hospital include rejection, infection, biliary complications, hypotension, recurrent disease, bone disease, nutrition and *de novo* cancer. Infections occur in most patients largely related to immunosuppression; chronic opportunistic infections usually occur from 4 weeks after transplant. Biliary strictures may also occur from 4 weeks after transplant. Acute liver rejection is rarely seen after the initial 6 months. Chronic rejection usually occurs 6 weeks to 9 months after transplant; there is progressive cholestasis and diagnosis is best made by liver biopsy. Bone disease and ectopic calcification may occur some months after transplant.

**Table 6-23.** *Causes of Fever in the Outpatient with a Liver Transplant*

Biliary tract (stricture and cholangitis)
Pneumonia (e.g., pneumocystis, bacterial, fungal)
Urinary tract sepsis
Hepatitis (acute or recurrent)
Central nervous system infection (especially fungal)
Viral infection (e.g., cytomegalovirus, herpes, varicella-zoster)

6. Ask about current medications and related complications with their use. Cyclosporin may induce cholestasis (dose-dependent), hypertension, nephrotoxicity. toxicity, gum hypertrophy, fits (controlled by phenytoin which itself induces cyclosporin metabolism) and central nervous system effects including tremor and central pontine myelinosis. Patients with a low serum cholesterol level are at increased risk of central nervous system toxicity. Steroids in high doses may induce a number of problems including aseptic necrosis of long bones, cataracts and psychosis. Enquire about drug compliance.
7. Ask about the specific complications of immunosuppression. Systemic and local infection are frequent problems and can be rapidly fatal if not treated aggressively. Opportunistic infections include *Pneumocystis carinii* and Candida. Cytomegalovirus infection remains a major problem. Try to find out tactfully whether there has been any problem with malignancy. Skin cancers and lymphomas (especially in the central nervous system) are increased with immunosuppression.

## The Examination (p. 165)

The pretransplant patient should be examined for signs of chronic liver disease and complications of liver disease.

The post-transplant patient should be examined for liver tenderness (e.g., acute rejection) and jaundice (e.g., vanishing bile ducts in chronic rejection, biliary stricture). Examine the chest for infection and the mouth for candidiasis. The temperature must be taken (Table 6-23). Examine the central nervous system (e.g., cyclosporin toxicity or cerebral infarction from perioperative hypotension or air embolism). Tap the spine for tenderness (e.g., vertebral collapse). Take the blood pressure (hypertension may occur at anytime after transplant; it is often caused by cyclosporin).

## Investigations and treatment

Pretransplant patients need tests to confirm the diagnosis, determine current liver synthetic function (e.g., serum albumin, prothrombin time) and rule out contraindications. Ultrasound and CT scan are routine. In patients with possible or definite malignancy, metastases must be sought. The hepatic arterial tree, portal vein and inferior vena cava need to be visualized by angiography. The bile ducts should be visualized by ERCP (or percutaneous cholangiography if ERCP fails). Psychiatric evaluation is important.

Routine outpatient monitoring after transplant should include blood count, electrolytes, renal and liver function tests and trough cyclosporin levels. Remember drug interactions with cyclosporin. Hypertension should be treated. Diseases that can recur in the graft include hepatitis B and C, Budd–Chiari syndrome and primary biliary cirrhosis.

# HAEMOLYTIC ANAEMIA

This is an uncommon but important long case. It is usually a diagnostic problem. Coombs' positive haemolytic anaemia may be the one most often encountered in the examination.

## The History

1. Presenting symptoms
   Ask about the symptoms of anaemia (e.g., fatigue, shortness of breath on exertion) and whether the patient has noticed or been told about jaundice.
2. Determine if there is a history of known haemolytic episodes. Onset at an early age or a family history suggests an intrinsic red cell defect (e.g., hereditary spherocytosis, sickle cell anaemia).
3. Ask about symptoms of connective tissue disease. Joint pain or swelling may also occur in acute sickle cell crises and especially affect the knees and elbows. Refractory leg ulcers occur in hereditary spherocytosis and sickle cell syndromes. Systemic lupus erythematosus is associated with warm antibody immunohaemolytic anaemia.
4. A history of pain in the abdomen, back and elsewhere suggests sickle cell anaemia or paroxysmal nocturnal haemoglobinuria. Congenital haemolytic anaemias can result in pigment gallstones that can cause acute cholecystitis; these episodes can be confused with acute crises.
5. Ask about neurological problems. Spinal cord lesions can occur with hereditary spherocytosis. Acute sickle cell crisis can also result in neurological impairment, particularly stroke. In thrombotic thrombocytopenic purpura there are often fluctuating neurological abnormalities. Tertiary syphilis may cause paroxysmal cold haemoglobinuria.
6. List all drugs that have been taken, e.g., alpha-methyldopa, penicillin and quinidine can cause warm antibody immunohaemolytic anaemia, while antimalarials, sulphonamides and nitrofurantoin cause haemolysis in subjects deficient in glucose 6-phosphate dehydrogenase.
7. Inquire about any operations, particularly heart valve replacement (10% of those with artificial aortic valve prostheses have significant haemolysis; this is less with mitral valve prostheses as the pressure gradient is lower). Severe haemolysis in these patients suggests a paravalvular leak.

8. Determine the patient's ethnic background, e.g., Greeks or Italians may inherit beta-thalassaemia trait, while black people may have glucose 6-phosphate dehydrogenase (G6PD) deficiency.

## The Examination (p. 182)

A careful haematopoietic system examination is required. The characteristic 'chipmunk' facies in a young person with thalassaemia is due to maxillary marrow hyperplasia and frontal bossing. Look for pallor and icterus. Examine the heart for a valve prosthesis or severe aortic stenosis (traumatic haemolysis). Profound anaemia may be associated with high output cardiac failure. An iron overload state in thalassaemia major from repeated transfusions may cause skin pigmentation, cardiac failure and hepatomegaly.

Carefully palpate for the spleen; splenomegaly from any cause (Table 8-19, p. 180) may result in haemolysis. Lymphadenopathy may indicate lymphoma (associated with warm or cold antibody haemolysis) or chronic lymphocytic leukaemia or infectious mononucleosis (cold agglutinin haemolysis). Signs of chronic liver disease should be noted—in severe cirrhosis spur-cell (acanthocyte) anaemia is occasionally observed. Look for focal neurological signs. Look in the fundi—retinal detachment, retinal infarcts and vitreous haemorrhages can be manifestations of sickle cell anaemia while Kayser-Fleischer rings may be present in the cornea in haemolysis caused by Wilson's disease.

Joint swelling and tenderness and occasionally aseptic necrosis of bone (e.g., neck of femur) also occur in sickle cell anaemia; bony infarcts may become infected (e.g., salmonella osteomyelitis). Look for leg ulceration. Note any signs of systemic lupus erythematosus (p. 97). Test the urine—urobilinogen may be present with haemolysis, it may be dark from haemosiderin or haemoglobin in severe haemolysis, and the sediment may be abnormal (e.g., thrombotic thombocytopenic purpura). Fever may occur with septicaemia or malaria-associated haemolysis, with acute crises in sickle cell anaemia and in thrombotic thombocytopenic purpura.

## Investigations

It is important to confirm that haemolysis is present, exclude intravascular haemolysis and perform tests to determine the aetiology. Ask for the results of a blood count, reticulocyte count, serum bilirubin and lactate dehydrogenase. Haemolysis is likely to be present if there is a normochromic normocytic anaemia with an increased reticulocyte count (but reticulocytes also occur with blood loss or partially treated anaemia) and release of red blood cell components (increased unconjugated bilirubin and, more variably, lactate dehydrogenase). In thalassaemia the anaemia is often hypochromic and microcytic. If there is doubt, the definitive test for haemolysis is a red cell survival study (using $^{51}$Cr-tagged red cells). Intravascular haemolysis is documented by the presence of methaemalbumin in the plasma and less often haemoglobin in the urine; usually serum haptoglobin is absent, and haemosiderin is present in the urine.

The history and physical examination may have provided hints about the likely aetiology. The blood film usually shows polychromasia; it may show other red cell changes (Table 6-24). If a congenital intracorpuscular defect seems unlikely, ask for a Coombs' test next to determine if the anaemia is immunohaemolytic. The polyspecific direct Coombs' test measures the ability of anti-IgG and anti-C3 to agglutinate the patient's red blood cells. 'Warm' antibodies react at body temperature and may occur with lymphoma (usually non-Hodgkin's), chronic lymphocytic leukaemia, systemic lupus erythematosus, drugs, or be idiopathic. 'Cold' reactive antibodies are precipitated by exposure to cold—cold agglutinin disease (IgM antibodies) may occur acutely with infectious mononucleosis or mycoplasma infection, and chronically may be due to lymphoma or be idiopathic; paroxysmal cold haemoglobinuria (IgG antibodies) is rare.

If the haemoglobinuria occurs usually at night and there is pancytopenia and venous thrombosis, paroxysmal noctural haemoglobinuria should be strongly suspected. Here the neutrophil alkaline phosphatase score is low, and the sucrose lysis and acid haemolysis (Ham's) test are usually postive; the red cell acetylcholinesterase is also decreased. Tests for haemolysis due to other causes are presented in Table 6-24.

## Treatment

This depends on the underlying disease process which should be reversed if possible (e.g., drug withdrawal) (Table 6-24). Steroids are useful in immunohaemolytic anaemia. Splenectomy is virtually curative in hereditary spherocytosis and may be useful in selected patients with massive splenomegaly, immunohaemolytic anaemia, certain haemoglobinopathies and enzymopathies, and spur-cell anaemia. Transfusion is not usually indicated unless there is symptomatic anaemia with a haemoglobin level less than 90g/L; it may exacerbate haemolysis.

# POLYCYTHAEMIA

The myeloproliferative disorders (Table 6-25) occur frequently in the Fellowship examination. They present a diagnostic and management problem. Polycythaemia rubra vera is the commonest myeloproliferative disease encountered. This disease occurs in later middle life and is more common in males. Secondary causes of polycythaemia must be excluded.

## The History

The patient will probably know the diagnosis. If you suspect polycythaemia ask about:

1. Symptoms of polycythaemia:
   (a) vascular effects, e.g., transient ischaemic episodes, angina, peripheral vascular disease (thrombosis);
   (b) bleeding from the nose;

**Table 6-24.** *Haemolytic Anaemia*

| Classification | Peripheral Blood Morphology | Diagnostic Test | Treatment |
|---|---|---|---|
| **Extracorpuscular** | | | |
| 1. Immune Haemolysis<br>　a. 'Warm' antibody<br>　　i) autoimmune<br>　　　(lymphoma,<br>　　　connective<br>　　　tissue disease,<br>　　　idiopathic)<br>　　ii) drug induced | Spherocytes | Coombs'<br>(antiglobulin) test;<br>differential Coombs'<br>test (IgG,<br>complement) | Autoimmune: clinically<br>significant haemolysis—<br>steroids; if steroids not<br>tolerated or do not<br>control disease—<br>splenectomy; if<br>still refractory—<br>azathioprine,<br>cyclophosphamide or<br>danazol<br>Drugs: discontinue |
| 　b) 'Cold' antibody<br>　　i) cold agglutinin<br>　　　(post-Infectious,<br>　　　lymphoma,<br>　　　idiopathic) | Red cell<br>agglutination<br>in cold | Cold agglutinins<br>Coombs' test—C3<br>on red cell surface<br>Anti-I (e.g.,<br>mycoplasma) or<br>anti-i (e.g., infectious<br>mononucleosis) | Maintain warm<br>environment;<br>immunosuppressives<br>only if severe disease |
| 2. Mechanical Haemolysis<br>　a) Microangiopathic<br>　　(DIC, TTP,<br>　　vasculitis, etc.) | Schizocytes,<br>microspherocytes | Evidence of<br>intravascular<br>haemolysis, evidence<br>of underlying disease<br>state | Microangiopathic TTP:<br>plasmaphaeresis |
| 　b) Heart valve | | | Heart valve: correct<br>iron deficiency; replace<br>valve if indicated |
| 　c) 'March<br>　　haemoglobinuria'<br>　　(e.g., marathon<br>　　runners) | | | March haemoglobinuria:<br>no specific therapy |
| 3. Infection<br>　a) Septicaemia<br>　b) Parasitic,<br>　　e.g., malaria | Spherocytes,<br>fragments,<br>intraerythrocyte<br>parasites | Blood cultures, thin<br>and thick smears | Treat infection |
| 4. Acquired Membrane Abnormalities<br>　a) Cirrhosis | Spur-cells<br>(acanthocytes) | Liver function tests,<br>etc., | Splenectomy if severe<br>haemolysis |
| 　b) Uraemia | Burr cells<br>(echinocytes) | Renal function tests | Treat renal failure<br>Correct iron deficiency |
| 　c) Paroxysmal<br>　　nocturnal<br>　　haemoglobinuria | Spherocytes,<br>microcytes | Acid serum lysis test,<br>sucrose lysis test,<br>decreased red cell<br>acetylcholinesterase,<br>deficiency of DAF in<br>red cell membrane | Steroid or androgen<br>may reduce haemolysis<br>Transfuse with washed<br>red cells |

*Table 6-24 (Continued)*

| Classification | Peripheral Blood Morphology | Diagnostic Test | Treatment |
|---|---|---|---|
| **Intracorpuscular** | | | |
| 1. Haemoglobinopathies | | | |
|   a) amino acid substitutions e.g., sickle cell | Sickle forms, hypochromic | Sickle preparation, Hgb electrophoresis | Detect infection early and treat, maintain adequate folic acid levels, acute crises—analgesia, oxygen if hypoxic |
|   b) Thalassaemias— beta thalassaemia alpha thalassaemia | Microcytic, target cells, tear drops | Hgb $A_2$ and F levels, globin synthesis study, gene mapping, family study of Hgbs | Beta thalassaemia major—supportive: transfusion, iron chelating therapy |
|   c) HgbH disease: inherited or acquired (myeloproliferative, myelodysplastic) | Heinz bodies on incubation | Hgb electrophoresis, brilliant cresyl blue preparation | HgbH—folic acid, avoid oxidant drugs, treat underlying disease |
| 2. Inherited Membrane Abnormalities e.g., spherocytosis | Spherocytes | Osmotic fragility (increased), red cell membrane protein study | Splenectomy corrects the anaemia |
| 3. Metabolic Abnormalities e.g., G6PD deficiency | 'Bite' cells, spherocytes | G6PD assay, G6PD electrophoresis | Prevent haemolytic episodes (avoid oxidant drugs, fava beans) |

Hgb = haemoglobin; HgbH = haemoglobin H; DAF = decay accelerating factors; TTP = thrombotic thrombocytopenic purpura; G6PD = glucose 6-phosphate dehydrogenase; DIC = disseminated intravascular coagulation.

**Table 6-25.** *Myeloproliferative Disorders*

1. Polycythaemia rubra vera
2. Myelofibrosis
3. Essential thrombocythaemia
4. Chronic myelogenous leukaemia

    (c) symptoms of peptic ulceration (increased 4 to 5 times in polycythaemia rubra vera);

    (d) abdominal pain or discomfort from gross splenomegaly or urate stones;

    (e) pruritus after showering;

    (f) gout.

2. Symptoms due to disease causing secondary polycythaemia (Table 6-26), e.g., chronic respiratory diseases, chronic cardiac diseases or congenital heart

**Table 6-26.** *Causes of Polycythaemia*

---

**Absolute Polycythaemia (increased red cell mass)**
1. Primary—polycythaemia rubra vera
2. Secondary polycythaemia
   a) Increased erythropoietin:
      i)   renal disease, e.g., polycystic disease, hydronephrosis, tumour
      ii)  hepatoma
      iii) cerebellar haemangioma
      iv) uterine myoma
      v)   virilizing syndromes (Table 8-38)
      vi) Cushing's syndrome
      vii) phaeochromocytoma
   b) Hypoxic states (erythopoietin secondarily increased):
      i)   chronic lung disease
      ii)  sleep apnoea
      iii) cyanotic congenital heart disease
      iv) abnormal haemoglobins (high affinity variants)
      v)   carbon monoxide poisoning

**Relative Polycythaemia (decreased plasma volume)**
1. Dehydration
2. Smokers' polycythaemia—carboxyhaemoglobinaemia (erythrocyte mass also increased)
3. Stress polycythaemia—Gaisbock's disease (? a distinct entity)

---

    diseases, renal diseases (especially polycystic kidneys, hydronephrosis or carcinoma).
3. Investigations performed and how the diagnosis was made, e.g., red cell mass measurement, blood counts, liver-spleen scan, and renal, pulmonary and cardiac investigations.
4. The treatment initiated, e.g., phlebotomy (how often and for how long), radio-active phosphorus, treatment of renal, pulmonary or cardiac disease.
5. Resolution of symptoms with treatment.
6. Social problems related to chronic disease.

# The Examination (P. 182)

Look at the patient. Note plethora, the state of hydration, cyanosis and any Cushingoid (p. 190) features.

    Examine the hands for nicotine stains, clubbing and signs of peripheral vascular disease. Note any gouty tophi. Look for scratch marks and bruising on the arms and take the blood pressure (for phaeochromocytoma) lying and standing.

    Look at the eyes for injected conjunctivae and examine the fundi for hyper-viscosity changes. Examine the tongue for central cyanosis.

    Examine the cardiovascular system for signs of cyanotic congenital heart disease if appropriate (p. 155), and the respiratory system for signs of chronic lung disease (p. 54).

Examine the abdomen for hepatomegaly (hepatoma must be excluded) and splenomegaly, which occurs in 80% of cases of polycythaemia rubra vera, but not in secondary polycythaemia. Palpate for renal masses (polycystic kidneys, hydronephrosis, carcinoma). Rarely, uterine fibromas may be found, or very rarely virilization may be noted. Epigastric tenderness may indicate a possible peptic ulcer but is not an accurate sign.

Look at the legs for scratch marks (pruritus may be secondary to elevated plasma histamine), gout and evidence of peripheral vascular disease. Auscultate over the cerebellar regions for a bruit (cerebellar haemangioblastoma). Note any upper motor neurone signs (cerebrovascular disease due to thrombosis or the hyperviscosity syndrome) (p. 233).

Check the urine for evidence of renal disease.

## Investigations

Confirm the presence of polycythaemia and establish whether this is primary or secondary.

1. Full blood count. In polycythaemia rubra vera the following are increased: haemoglobin value, haematocrit value, red cell count, white cell count (including the absolute basophil count), platelet count, and more variably the neutrophil alkaline phosphatease (NAP) score. The ESR is very low in both primary and secondary polycythaemia.
2. Confirm absolute polycythaemia is present with an elevated red blood cell mass (chromium-51-labelled red blood cells) and usually a normal or sometimes increased plasma volume (isotope-labelled albumin).
3. Bone marrow. In polycythaemia rubra vera there is significant panhyperplasia and iron stores are often reduced, but in secondary polycythaemia the bone marrow is usually normal.
4. Vitamin $B_{12}$ binding capacity. The total $B_{12}$ level is elevated in 75% of cases of polycythaemia rubra vera. The $B_{12}$ level is raised due to increased transcobalamin I and III made by the neutrophils, which have an increased turnover.
5. If in doubt, check the arterial blood gases (in polycythaemia rubra vera 80% of patients have a saturation >92% and almost all have a saturation ≥88%).
6. Rule out renal disease with intravenous pyelography if indicated.
7. Serum erythropoietin is usually substantially reduced or absent in polycythaemia rubra vera and elevated in secondary polycythaemia.

## Treatment

The aim is to lower the haematocrit value at least below 0.45 and maintain it at this level. Most patients die of thrombosis. Untreated cases have a median survival of two years. This is extended to ten years with phlebotomy alone.

Polycythaemia rubra vera should be treated by phlebotomy. Radioactive phosphorus ($^{32}$P) irradiates the bone marrow and is easy to use and effective, but it increases the incidence of acute myeloid leukaemia and should be avoided in patients under the age of 70 years. Alkylating agents (e.g., busulphan) must be monitored closely for the same reason and should not be given routinely. Pruritus may respond to antihistamines and hyperuricaemia should be treated with allopurinol. Aspirin should be reserved for thrombotic events in patients with thrombocytosis as bleeding is a more common complication. Symptomatic organomegaly may respond to local irradiation or hydroxyurea. Secondary polycythaemia is treated by removal of the cause, and phlebotomy if the haematocrit exceeds 0.55.

# LYMPHOMA

These diseases provide complicated diagnostic and management problems. Treatment in expert units is important as some patients are cured.

Hodgkin's disease (Table 6-27) presents either with discrete, rubbery, painless nodules, or with generalized symptoms (fever, night sweats, weight loss and sometimes pruritus). Mediastinal adenopathy usually occurs in young people with nodular sclerosing disease. Older people with generalized symptoms, in whom the only enlarged nodes may be in the abdomen, often have lymphocyte-depleted Hodgkin's disease.

Non-Hodgkin's lymphoma (Table 6-27) usually presents as localized or generalized painless adenopathy with or without hepatosplenomegaly. It may also present with just an abdominal mass. Waldeyer's ring involvement is more common in non-Hodgkin's than in Hodgkin's disease. Systemic symptoms are less common in non-Hodgkin's lymphoma. In nodular lymphoma, lymphadenopathy has often been present for a long time.

## The History

1. Presenting symptoms, e.g., nodes, systemic symptoms, bone pain due to marrow infiltration or pathological fractures, spinal cord compression, splenic pain, alcohol-induced pain (rare).
2. History of infection (due to decreased cell-mediated immunity in Hodgkin's disease or depressed humoral immunity from chemotherapy or radiotherapy).
3. Investigations performed—particularly lymphangiography and staging laparotomy, CT scans and bilateral bone marrow aspirations and biopsies.
4. Treatment undertaken—an indication of the stage and type of disease. Ask about side effects of any treatment (e.g., mantle radiation can result in pneumonitis, hypothyroidism, pericarditis, myocardial fibrosis and spinal cord injury).
5. The prognosis given.
6. The social situation—dependent family members, social support, ability to work, etc.

## The Examination (p. 182)

Examine the haemopoietic system thoroughly. Attempt to stage the disease clinically (Table 6-28). Note any radiotherapy marks (and the field covered). Look for evidence of infection (e.g., herpes zoster).

**Table 6-27.**  *Histopathological Classification of Lymphoma*

**Hodgkin's Disease**
1. Lymphocyte predominant
2. Nodular sclerosing
3. Mixed cellularity
4. Lymphocyte depleted

**Non-Hodgkin's Lymphoma**
*Rappaport*
I   Favourable Prognosis Group
 1. Diffuse lymphocytic, well differentiated
 2. Nodular lymphocytic, poorly differentiated
 3. Nodular mixed

II  Intermediate Prognosis Group
 1. Nodular histiocytic
 2. Diffuse lymphocytic, poorly differentiated
 3. Diffuse mixed

III Unfavourable Prognosis Group
 1. Diffuse histiocytic
 2. Lymphoblastic convoluted/non-convoluted
 3. Diffuse undifferentiated

*International Working Formulation*
I   Low-Grade Lymphoma
 1. Small lymphocytic cell
 2. Follicular, mixed cleaved cell
 3. Follicular, mixed small cleaved and large cell

II  Intermediate-Grade Lymphoma
 1. Follicular large cell
 2. Diffuse small cleaved cell
 3. Diffuse mixed small cleaved cell
 4. Diffuse large cell

III High-Grade Lymphoma
 1. Large cell immunoblastic
 2. Lymphoblastic cell
 3. Small non-cleaved cell (Burkitt and non-Burkitt)

**Table 6-28.**  *Staging of Lymphoma—Ann Arbor Classification*

| | |
|---|---|
| Stage I | Disease confined to a single lymph node region or a single extralymphatic site(Ie) |
| Stage II | Disease confined to 2 or more lymph node regions on the same side of the diaphragm, plus or minus splenic involvement. |
| Stage III | Disease confined to lymph node regions on both sides of the diaphragm ($III_1$ = upper abdomen; $III_2$ = lower abdomen), with or without localized involvement of the spleen (IIIs), other extralymphatic organ or site (IIIe), or both |
| Stage IV | Diffuse disease of one or more extralymphatic organs (with or without lymph node disease) |
| For any stage: | A. No symptoms<br>B. Fever, weight loss > 10% in 6 months or night sweats |

# Investigations

The first step is to obtain histological confirmation of disease. Ask to see the pathology report if lymph node biopsies have already been performed. Reed-Sternberg cells are *not* pathognomonic of Hodgkin's disease but may occur in infectious mononucleosis, other viral diseases and with other malignancies.

The next step is to stage the disease further. Ask for a full blood count and ESR, a bilateral bone marrow aspirate and trephine, liver function tests, chest X-ray film and abdominal and chest imaging (e.g., CT scan). In Hodgkin's disease, granulo-cytosis (sometimes with marked eosinophilia or a leukaemoid reaction), an ele-vated ESR, elevated haptoglobin levels and a mildy elevated alkaline phosphatase level are often present but may *not* indicate widespread disease. Lymphangio-graphy is less often done in Hodgkin's disease if the CT scan and other non-invasive investigations give normal results, but minimal nodal involvement can be missed if it is omitted. Staging laparotomy is often required, unless evidence of stage IV disease is already present. Re-staging after therapy to determine whether a complete remission has occurred is important.

# Treatment

## *Hodgkin's Disease*

Treatment depends on the stage of the disease. Histological type is less important here.

Stage IA, IIA, and III$_1$A: Radiotherapy

Stage III$_2$A, IIIB and IV: Combined chemotherapy, e.g., MOPP (nitrogen mustard, vincristine, procarbazine, prednisone).

Stage I or II with systemic symptoms (B), a large mediastinal mass, or contiguous extralymphatic extension (E): controversial (radiotherapy or chemotherapy)

Prognosis depends on the stage. In general, in:

Stage I, expect 85% to 95% 10 years' disease-free survival;
Stage II, expect 80% to 90% 10 years' disease-free survival;
Stage III and IV, expect 60% 10 years' disease-free survival.

## *Non-Hodgkin's Lymphoma*

Prognosis and treatment depend mainly on the histological type (particularly whether it is nodular or diffuse); most low-grade lymphomas are stage III or IV at presentation.

### *Low-grade Lymphoma*

Nodular low-grade lymphoma has a good prognosis for survival, but is not gen-erally curable. Commonly it presents as stage IVA.

For asymptomatic nodular lymphoma, no treatment is indicated.

For symptomatic nodular lymphoma, chlorambucil is the usual initial treatment.

For Stage I and II nodular lymphoma (uncommon), extended field radiation may be used in younger patients with curative intent, but they must be very carefully staged first.

### Intermediate and High-grade Lymphoma

Intermediate and high-grade lymphoma have a poor prognosis if untreated. Diffuse large-cell lymphoma and high-grade lymphomas are potentially curable with treatment.

    Stage I and II (uncommon): aggressive treatment to try for cure is essential, but careful staging must be carried out first.

    Stage III and IV:

(a) diffuse large cell lymphoma—combination chemotherapy, e.g., CHOP (cyclophosphamide, adriamycin, vincristine and prednisone);

(b) diffuse well-differentiated lymphocytic lymphoma—this is the most indolent type and prognosis is indistinguishable from that of chronic lymphocytic leukaemia; no treatment is required unless symptomatic;

(c) other diffuse types: these respond to chemotherapy, but disease-free survival is not improved.

# MULTIPLE MYELOMA

This is a disseminated malignant disease of plasma cells. It occurs in the elderly—the median age is 60 years—and more often in males. It can present as a diagnostic or management problem.

## The History

Ask about:

1. Presenting symptoms.
   (a) bone pain or pain with movement, particularly in the ribs or axial skeleton, and pathological fractures;
   (b) bacterial infection—particularly pneumonia (as the level of normal functional immunoglobulins is reduced);
   (c) symptoms of anaemia—due to bone marrow depression from infiltration, chronic disease, renal failure or treatment;
   (d) bleeding tendency—due to paraprotein inactivation of plasma procoagulants and reduced platelet function;
   (e) renal disease symptoms (due to hypercalcaemia, hyperuricaemia, tubular damage by light chains, therapy, urinary tract infection, contrast studies, plasma cell infiltration or amyloid) (p. 113);
   (f) hypercalcaemic symptoms due to bone lysis;
   (g) spinal cord compression (p. 239) or rarely diffuse sensorimotor neuropathy;
   (h) skin changes, e.g., pruritus, purpura, yellow skin, hypertrichosis (rare), erythema annulare (rare);
   (i) systemic amyloid deposition.

2. How the diagnosis was made.
3. Treatment
4. The social history, including dependents, work, etc.

## The Examination (p. 182)

Inspect the patient for signs of weight loss and general debility.

Examine the haemopoietic system. Pay particular attention to a search for bony tenderness. Kyphosis may be due to compression fractures. Note signs of anaemia and purpura. Look for skin rash. Note any signs of spinal cord compression. Check the urine analysis and temperature chart. Look for signs of infection (e.g., pulmonary consolidation).

## Investigations

Once the diagnosis is suspected, check the full blood count for anaemia and a raised ESR. Obtain a protein electrophoretogram (EPG) of serum and urine and also an immunoelectrophorectogram (IEPG). A monoclonal globulin peak is found in 99% of cases. In the urine, light chains are present in 50% to 75% (Bence-Jones proteinuria cannot be detected by dipstick urine analysis). The bone marrow must be examined for plasma cells.

Look at X-ray films of the skull, chest, pelvis and proximal long bones for lytic lesions, fractures and osteoporosis. Also check the serum calcium and urate levels and the renal function.

The three major diagnostic features of multiple myeloma are, in order of importance:

1. Production of serum paraprotein (50% are IgG, 33% IgA, 5% to 10% IgM, 10% only light chains, 1% nil)
2. Plasma cells in the bone marrow (>10% involvement is consistent with the diagnosis)
3. Bone destruction (lytic lesions).

Poor prognostic features include anaemia (haemoglobin <86g/L), hypercalcaemia, advanced lytic bone lesions, high M component production rates, an elevated creatinine level and an elevated serum beta$_2$ microglobulin level (which reflects the myeloma cell burden).

## Treatment

Irradiation is helpful for localized bone pain and spinal cord compression. Adequate hydration and bicarbonate for Bence-Jones proteinuria are important to prevent renal failure. Intravenous contrast material must be used cautiously and only with excellent hydration. Treat hypercalcaemia and bacterial infection. Avoid live vaccines.

Chemotherapy is indicated when patients are symptomatic or have rising myeloma protein levels or progressive lytic bone lesions. Melphalan and prednisone are

standard treatment; VMCP (vincristine, melphalan, cyclophosphamide and prednisone) is also useful.

Prognosis is poor. Forty months represent median survival. Secondary acute
leukaemia is being increasingly seen related to alkylating agent therapy.

## Differential Diagnosis

### Benign Monoclonal Gammopathy

A smaller IgG or IgA peak (<30g/L), normal serum immunoglobulin levels
and excretion of less than 100mg of Bence-Jones protein per day suggests this
diagnosis.

### Waldenström's Macroglobulinaemia

The EPG has a peak consisting of monoclonal IgM. These patients are generally
older than those with myeloma. The hyperviscosity syndrome is often present;
symptoms and signs include lassitude, confusion, bleeding, anaemia, infection,
lymphadenopathy, dilated retinal veins and perivenous haemorrhages, and (rarely)
renal failure. Lytic bone destruction is rare. An underlying lymphoproliferative
disorder may be present. Treatment with plasmapheresis is effective in removing
IgM paraprotein. Prednisone and chlorambucil are useful. Median survival is 4
years.

### Localized Myeloma

Only one plasma cell tumour is present. Solitary plasmacytomas often occur in the
nasopharynx or paranasal sinuses. The major complications of myeloma are absent. Only 50% of cases show a monoclonal peak. Local radiotherapy is the usual
treatment.

# RHEUMATOID ARTHRITIS

This is a very common long case. There are usually many physical signs. The
diagnosis is mostly straightforward. Management is often the major problem. The
peak incidence of rheumatoid arthritis is in the fourth decade, and it is 3 times as
common in women as in men. There is a familial incidence (HLA DR-4 is found
in 70% of patients).

## The History

Ask about:

1. When the diagnosis was made.
2. The presenting features (Table 6-29).
3. Initial treatment.
4. The disease progression.
5. The alterations in treatment over time and any complications encountered.
6. The non-articular features of the disease:
    (a) skin, e.g., Raynaud's phenomenon, leg ulcers;

**Table 6-29.** *Criteria for the Diagnosis of Rheumatoid Arthritis (≥4 of 7 criteria is diagnostic)*

1. Morning stiffness ≥6 weeks
2. Arthritis of 3 or more joint areas (soft tissue swelling or fluid for ≥6 weeks of PIP, MCP, wrist, elbow, knee, ankle, MTP joints)
3. Arthritis of hand joints ≥6 weeks (*not* DIP joint)
4. Symmetric arthritis ≥6 weeks (for joints defined in 2)
5. Rheumatoid nodules
6. Serum rheumatoid factor
7. X-ray changes of rheumatoid arthritis

N.B.  DIP = distal interphalangeal joint; PIP = proximal interphalangeal joint; MCP = metacarpophalangeal joint; MTP = metatarsophalangeal joint.

    (b) lungs, e.g., dyspnoea due to diffuse interstitial fibrosis or pleural effusion, pain due to pleuritis;

    (c) eyes, e.g., Sjögren's syndrome (dry eyes and mouth), scleritis, episcleritis or scleromalacia perforans, cataracts (due to steroids);

    (d) nervous system, e.g., peripheral neuropathy, mononeuritis multiplex, cord compression (due to cervical spine involvement or rheumatoid nodules), entrapment neuropathy (particularly carpal tunnel syndrome) (p. 237);

    (e) blood, e.g., anaemic symptoms due to chronic disease, iron deficiency (from blood loss), folate deficiency (diet); Felty's syndrome (rheumatoid arthritis with leukopenia and splenomegaly);

    (f) heart, e.g., chest pain due to pericarditis;

    (g) renal, e.g., infection, analgesic abuse, amyloid.

7. Drug complications:

    (a) aspirin, e.g., nausea, gastric erosions or ulcers causing bleeding, tinnitus;

    (b) non-steroidal anti-inflammatory drugs, e.g., acute ulceration, renal impairment;

    (c) gold, e.g., proteinuria, thrombocytopenia, rash, mouth ulcers or (rarely) enterocolitis or hepatitis;

    (d) penicillamine, e.g., nephrotic syndrome, thrombocytopenia, rashes, mouth ulcers, alteration in taste and (rarely) systemic lupus erythematosus, polymyositis, myasthenia gravis, Goodpasture's syndrome, or pulmonary infiltration;

    (e) steroids (p. 190);

    (f) immunosuppressive drugs, especially methotrexate.

8. The major current problem, e.g., decreasing hand power, paraesthesiae, etc.

9. Current activity of the disease. This can be assessed historically by asking about the number of joints that have recently been involved with active synovitis, the severity and duration of early morning stiffness (very important), the functional ability, change in weight and the degree of systemic ill health.

10. Social background, e.g., ability to cope at home, ability to climb steps,

independence in daily activities, ability to perform fine activities, the work environment, etc.
11. Family history.
12. Past medical history, especially of peptic ulceration, drug reactions or renal disease.

## The Examination (Figure 1)

A thorough general examination is important. In addition to assessing for synovitis in *every* joint, look particularly for the following:

1. General appearance—steroid complications (p. 190), weight.
2. The hands—including vasculitis and hand function (p. 200).
3. Arms—the elbow and shoulder joints, rheumatoid nodules and axillary nodal enlargement.
4. The face. The eyes for Sjögren's syndrome, scleritis, episcleritis, scleromalacia perforans, cataracts, anaemia and signs of hyperviscosity in the fundi. Enlarged parotid glands (Sjögren's syndrome). The mouth (dryness, dental caries, ulcers), hoarse voice, temporomandibular joint (crepitus).
   N.B. Rheumatoid arthritis does not cause iritis.
5. The neck—for signs of cervical spine involvement.
6. The chest. The heart (for pericarditis, conduction defects, aortic and mitral incompetence) (p. 135). The lungs (for pleural effusion, fibrosis, nodules, infarction, Caplan's syndrome) (p. 160).
7. The abdomen—for splenomegaly and epigastric tenderness (p. 165).
8. The hips and knees (p. 203).
9. The lower legs—for ulcers, calf swelling (ruptured Baker's cyst), neuropathy, mononeuritis multiplex and signs of cord compression (p. 230).
10. The feet (p. 204).
11. Urine analysis for protein and blood, and rectal examination for blood.

## Management

Consider the differential diagnosis of a deforming symmetrical chronic polyarthropathy:

1. Rheumatoid arthritis
2. Psoriatic arthropathy and other seronegative spondyloarthropathies
3. Chronic tophaceous gout (rarely symmetrical)
4. Primary generalized osteoarthritis
5. Infection, e.g., Lyme arthritis (very rare spirochaetal infection).

Remember the causes of arthritis plus nodules include:

1. Rheumatoid arthritis (seropositive)
2. Systemic lupus erythematosus—rare
3. Rheumatic fever (Jaccoud's arthritis)—very rare
4. Amyloid arthropathy (most usually in association with multiple myeloma).
   N.B. Gouty tophi and xanthoma may sometimes cause confusion.

**Figure 1.**  *Rheumatoid Arthritis*

GENERAL INSPECTION
  Cushingoid appearance
  Weight

HANDS (p. 200)

ARMS
  Entrapment neuropathy
    (e.g., carpal tunnel)
  Subcutaneous nodules
  Elbow joint
  Shoulder joint
  Axillary nodes

NECK
  Cervical spine
  Cervical nodes

CHEST
  Heart—Pericarditis, Valve lesions
  Lungs—Effusion, Fibrosis,
  Infarction, Infection, Nodules
    (and Caplan's syndrome)
  Tuberculosis (steroids)

ABDOMEN
  Splenomegaly (e.g., Felty's syndrome)
  Epigastric tenderness (drugs)
  Inguinal nodes

HIPS

KNEES (p. 203)

FACE
  Eyes—dry eyes (Sjögren's)—
    scleritis, episcleritis
  Scleromalacia perforans—anaemia—
  Cataract (steroids, chloroquine)—
  Fundi—hyperviscosity
  Face—parotids (Sjögren's)
  Mouth—dryness, ulcers, dental
    caries, temporomandibular joint
    (crepitus)

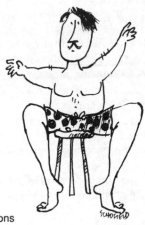

LOWER LIMBS
  Ulceration (vasculitis)
  Calf swelling (ruptured synovial cyst)
  Peripheral neuropathy
  Mononeuritis multiplex
  Cord compression

FEET (p. 204)

OTHER
  Urine: Protein, blood (drugs,
    vasculitis, infection, amyloidosis)
  Rectal examination (blood)

## Investigations

To support the diagnosis (remembering that this is primarily a clinical diagnosis):

1. Serological tests:
   (a) rheumatoid factor—70% of patients are seropositive.
   N.B. 100% are rheumatoid factor positive if they have nodules or Sjögren's syndrome;
   (b) antinuclear antibody (ANA)—positive results in about 20% of cases.
2. X-ray films of involved joints. Changes to look for are:
   (a) soft tissue swelling;
   (b) joint space narrowing;
   (c) joint erosions;
   (d) juxta-articular osteoporosis.

To assess the activity of the disease:

1. Progressive erosions on serial X-ray films.
2. Erythrocyte sedimentation rate (ESR). Remember the differential diagnosis of a raised ESR in rheumatoid arthritis includes:
   (a) active disease;
   (b) amyloidosis;
   (c) infection;
   (d) Sjögren's syndrome.
3. Anaemia—the severity of normochromic anaemia usually correlates with activity.
4. Rheumatoid factor titre—the higher the titre the more likely the patient is to have extra-articular features. It does *not* correlate with activity of arthritis.

## Treatment

This should include:

1. Education.
2. Physiotherapy including exercise and splinting of joints to prevent deformity.
3. Occupational therapy.
4. Drug treatment should begin with a non-steroidal anti-inflammatory drug. If there is a failure to decrease inflammation after 4 to 8 weeks switching to a different chemical class may be helpful. With active progressive disease, suppressive treatment using gold (parenteral or oral) is often desirable. With parenteral gold therapy—always give a test dose first (10mg) and then 50mg weekly until 1000mg is reached, then decrease the frequency of the injection over several months to 50mg once monthly. On this regimen 40% of patients will have a remission and 30% will show improvement. Oral gold may be less effective. Monitor regularly for proteinuria (>500mg/24hours) and bone marrow depression (leukopenia or thrombocytopenia) which are indicators for cessation of therapy. D-penicillamine use is restricted by complications of renal toxicity and bone marrow depression. Local steroid injections are helpful for acute involvement of a joint, but only give temporary relief.

Low-dose steroid treatment may retard joint damage. The main indications for steroid use are:

1. Vasculitic complications of rheumatoid arthritis (where high doses are needed).
2. Severe progressive disease until suppressive treatment with gold becomes effective (low dose).
3. Low-dose treatment in the elderly may be justifiable.

Methotrexate, 7.5mg taken *one* day a week, can be used for severe disease, especially when other therapy has failed; improvement is seen in 1 to 2 months, but myelosuppression, pneumonitis and liver disease are potential complications.

# SYSTEMIC LUPUS ERYTHEMATOSUS

This multi-system disorder occurs usually in patients between 20 and 40 years of age. Females are more often affected than males (7:1) and there is an increased incidence in families. It presents diagnostic problems as well as long-term management problems.

## The History

Ask about:

1. Presenting symptoms (Table 6-30):
    (a) general symptoms—malaise (100%), weight loss (60%), nausea and vomiting (50%), thrombosis of veins or arteries (15%);
    (b) musculoskeletal symptoms (95%)—arthralagia and arthritis, myositis;
    (c) dermatological symptoms (85%)—skin rash, alopecia;
    (d) fever (77%);
    (e) neurological symptoms (60%)—delirium, dementia, convulsions, chorea, neuropathy, symptoms resembling multiple sclerosis;
    (f) renal tract symptoms (50%)—haematuria, oedema, renal failure;
    (g) respiratory tract symptoms (45%)—pleurisy;
    (h) cardiovascular symptoms (40%)—pericarditis;
    (i) haematological symptoms (50%)—lymphadenopathy, anaemia;
    (j) thrombophlebitis, recurrent abortions or fetal death in utero (suggests lupus anticoagulant);
    (k) Sjögren's syndrome.
2. Any drug history, e.g., procainamide, hydralazine (Table 6-31).
3. Any treatment given and any complications of treatment.
4. Family history.
5. Social background.

## The Examination (Figure 2)

Inspect the patient for weight loss, Cushingoid (p. 190) appearance (because of steroid treatment) and general mental state.

Look at the hands (p. 200) for vasculitis and rash (e.g., photosensitivity, diffuse maculopapular rash). Also look for Raynaud's phenomenon and arthropathy

**Figure 2.**   *Systemic Lupus Erythematosus (SLE)*

GENERAL INSPECTION
  Cushingoid
  Weight
  Mental state

HEAD
  Alopecia, lupus hairs
  Eyes—scleritis, cytoid lesions, etc.
  Mouth—ulcers, infection
  Nose—nasoseptal perforation
  Rash, e.g., butterfly
  Cranial nerve lesions
  Cervical adenopathy

HANDS
  Vasculitis
  Rash
  Arthropathy

CHEST
  Cardiovascular system—endocarditis
  Respiratory system—pleural effusion,
    pleurisy, pulmonary fibrosis,
    collapse or infection

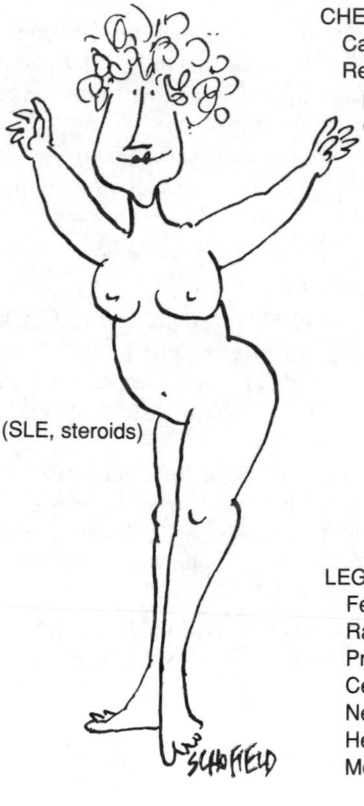

ABDOMEN
  Hepatosplenomegaly
  Tenderness

ARMS
  Livedo reticularis
  Purpura
  Proximal myopathy (SLE, steroids)

HIPS
  Aseptic necrosis

LEGS
  Feet—red soles, small joint synovitis
  Rash
  Proximal myopathy
  Cerebellar ataxia
  Neuropathy (uncommon)
  Hemiplegia
  Mononeuritis multiplex

OTHER
  Urine analysis (proteinuria)
  Blood pressure (hypertension)
  Temperature chart

(synovitis possibly in a rheumatoid arthritis distribution—uncommon). Look at the forearms for livedo reticularis and purpura due to vasculitis or thrombocyto penia. Test for proximal myopathy due to actual disease or steroid treatment.

Inspect the head. Look for alopecia. Lupus hairs are characteristic; they occur above the forehead and are short, broken hairs that grow back quickly after hair loss. Look at the eyes for scleritis, episcleritis and for pale conjunctivae from anaemia, and look at the fundi for cytoid lesions (hard exudates secondary to vasculitis). Look in the mouth for ulcers and infection. Note any facial rash (butterfly rash, discoid lupus or diffuse maculopapular rashes). Feel the cervical and axillary nodes.

Examine the chest. In the cardiovascular system note signs of pericarditis or murmurs (Libman-Sacks endocarditis is very rarely diagnosed in life). In the respiratory system note signs of pleural effusion, pleurisy, pulmonary fibrosis or atelectasis (p. 160).

Examine the abdomen for splenomegaly (usually mild) and hepatomegaly.

Examine the hips for signs of aseptic necrosis and examine for proximal weakness in the legs, cerebellar ataxia and hemiplegia.

Also examine for neuropathy (mainly sensory) and mononeuritis multiplex (pp. 234, 235) as well as thrombophlebitis and leg ulceration.

Look at the urine analysis (for evidence of renal disease) and take the blood pressure (may be elevated in renal disease). Also look at the temperature chart (for fever indicating active disease or secondary infection).

## Investigations

Diagnosis depends on a combination of the symptoms, signs and laboratory test results (Tables 6-30 to 6-33).

Patients who do not fit the criteria may have another connective tissue disease.

Mixed connective tissue disease (MCTD) is an overlap syndrome between systemic lupus erythematosus, scleroderma and polymyositis. The diagnosis is suggested by the overlapping clinical features of these syndromes and the presence of characteristic antibodies—to nuclear ribonucleoprotein (nRNP) which is one of the extractable nuclear antigens. Anti-nRNP is present in high titre and produces a speckled pattern on fluorescent antibody testing in patients with MCTD.

The important laboratory tests in systemic lupus erythematosus are haematological and serological.

### Haematological Tests

Anaemia—normochromic normocytic and related to the chronic inflammatory processes—is very common. Immune haemolytic anaemia is less common and the Coombs test then gives a positive result (p. 80).

Leukopenia occurs in over half the patients and may be due to antibody directed against leukocytes.

Clotting factor deficiencies are infrequent and are related to antibodies to factors VII, IX or X.

The lupus anticoagulant is found in about 10% of cases. Characteristically there

**Table 6-30.** *The American Rheumatism Association Criteria for Systemic Lupus Erythematosus 1982 (revised)*

**Clinical features**
1. Malar rash
2. Discoid lupus
3. Photosensitivity
4. Oral ulcers
5. Arthritis (non-erosive)
6. Pericarditis or pleuritis
7. Seizures or psychosis or an organic mental syndrome or neuropathy (e.g., cranial nerve) or ocular field defects, hemiparesis, aphasia or movement disorder, tremor

**Laboratory features**
8. Proteinuria (more than 0.5g/day) or cellular casts
9. Haemolytic anaemia or leucopenia or lymphopenia or thrombocytopenia
10. Positive antinuclear antibody (ANA)
11. Antibody to dsDNA or Sm (relatively specific) or LE cells or false-positive results in serological tests for syphilis

N.B. Four manifestations out of the 11 must be present serially or simultaneously (but are NOT diagnostic).

**Table 6-31.** *Drugs Inducing Systemic Lupus Erythematosus*

1. Procainamide (most patients are ANA positive within 1 year; 15% to 20% develop SLE)
2. Hydralazine (most patients are ANA positive within 1 year; 5% to 10% develop SLE)
3. Isoniazid*
4. Methyldopa*
5. Penicillamine*
6. Chlorpromazine*
7. Anticonvulsants*, particularly phenytoin (not sodium valproate)

N.B. There is an increased incidence of drug-induced lupus in slow acetylators who will develop a positive ANA and clinical manifestations sooner than rapid acetylators. Drug-induced lupus is more common in the elderly because of the more frequent use of drugs in this group. There is usually no renal or nervous system disease, no antibody to double-stranded DNA and improvement *may* occur if the drug is withdrawn.

* Rarely cause overt SLE, but ANA is commonly positive

is a prolonged PTTK which is not corrected by the addition of normal plasma. It is associated with thrombosis rather than bleeding.

Thrombocytopenia occurs in 15% of cases and is associated with antiplatelet antibodies.

## Immunological Tests

The characteristic abnormalities are the presence of autoantibodies (Tables 6-32, 6-33). Antibodies to nuclear antigens (ANA) are present in 99% of cases. The antigens involved include single and double stranded DNA, ribonucleoprotein and Sm antigen (an acidic nuclear protein). Many antibodies persist even when the disease is quiet. Antibodies to double-stranded DNA are the most specific for systemic lupus erythematosus and are therefore the most useful diagnostically.

**Table 6-32.** *Antinuclear Antibody (ANA) Patterns*

1. Rim or shaggy pattern—antibody to double-stranded DNA = SLE (50% to 60%)
2. Homogeneous pattern—antibody to deoxyribonucleoprotein = connective tissue disease, including SLE
3. Speckled pattern—antibody to extractable nuclear antigen = SLE or scleroderma or mixed connective tissue disease
4. Nucleolar pattern—antibody to RNA found especially in scleroderma

**Table 6-33.** *Antibodies Associated With Connective Tissue Diseases*

| Disease | Antibodies Associated |
|---------|----------------------|
| Systemic Lupus Erythematosus (SLE) | Anti-single-stranded DNA (not specific) |
| | Anti-double-stranded DNA (50% to 60%) |
| | Antibody to extractable nuclear antigen |
| | Anti-Sm (30%) |
| | Anti-RNP (30% in low titre) |
| | Anti-SS-A (30%) |
| | Anti-SS-B (15%) |
| | Anti-histone (drug-induced SLE: 95%) |
| Scleroderma and CREST | Anti-centromere (CREST: 70%; scleroderma: 10%) |
| | Anti-nucleolar, Anti Sci-70 (scleroderma 40%) |
| | Anti-RNP, Anti-SS-A (scleroderma occasionally in low titre) |
| Sjögren's | Anti-SS-A (70%), Anti SS-B (60%) |
| Mixed Connective Tissue Disease (MCTD) | Anti-RNP (100%) |
| | Anti-SS-A (occasionally in low titre) |
| Polymyositis and Dermatomyositis | Anti-PM1 (polymyositis: 50%; dermatomyositis: 10%) |

Complement abnormalities are usual during exacerbations of the disease with reduction in total haemolytic complement (CH50) and in the components of the classical pathway (C3 and C4). The finding of high levels of anti-ds DNA and lower complement levels is usually associated with active disease and especially renal involvement.

Positive rheumatoid factor occurs in 10% of cases at low titre. Skin biopsy of involved and uninvolved skin in SLE can be helpful; positive immunofluorescence of the basement membrane in involved skin occurs in 95% of patients and in non-involved skin in 50% of cases (the latter is called a positive lupus band test).

## Treatment

Current work suggests that appropriate treatment to suppress exacerbations of SLE will prolong life.

Arthralgias, myalgia and fever respond to rest and salicylates or non-steroidal anti-inflammatory drugs. Exposure to sunlight should be avoided and sunscreen should be used. Hydroxychloroquine is useful in the management of arthritis and

① NSAIDs
② Hydroxychloroquine
③ Steroids
④ Anticoagulants
⑤ Immunosuppressive

skin rash. Raynaud's phenomenon may respond to nifedipine or other medications (p. 105). Steroids are indicated for central nervous system involvement, pericarditis, myocarditis, pleurisy, severe haemolytic anaemia, worrying leukopenia and thrombocytopenia. Use of high initial doses with gradual reduction once improvement occurs is the proper method of treatment. Hypercoagulability may be treated by anticoagulants.

Management of renal disease is difficult. Renal biopsy usually shows abnormalities, but often only mild changes. Renal biopsy is indicated early if there is any clinical or biochemical evidence of renal disease or the urine sediment is abnormal. Four groups of biopsy abnormality can be identified: mesangial proliferation, focal glomerulonephritis, diffuse proliferation and membranous proliferation. Mesangial proliferation has the best prognosis; disease is unlikely to progress. Diffuse proliferative glomerulonephritis has the worst prognosis and aggressive treatment (e.g., high-dose steroids plus a cytotoxic drug) is recommended. Membranous proliferation has a low rate of response to treatment. Azathioprine is indicated as a steroid-sparing agent. Cyclophosphamide is a more toxic alternative. Intermittent pulses of cyclophosphamide may be helpful. These agents are particularly indicated in active glomerulonephritis. Plasmaphaeresis is sometimes used in severe disease but is not of proven benefit.

The prognosis of systemic lupus erythematosus is generally good. There is a 75% 10-year survival; the major causes of death are infections and renal failure.

Remember that post-partum exacerbations of lupus may occur.

# SYSTEMIC SCLEROSIS (SCLERODERMA)

This is a progressive disease of multiple organs. Although a rare disease, it crops up commonly in examinations. It is more common in women (2:1).

## The History

Ask about:

1. Presenting symptoms:
   (a) dermatological symptoms—Raynaud's phenomenon, tight skin, disability from sclerodactyly;
   (b) arthritis—arthropathy in a rheumatoid distribution, carpal tunnel symptoms;
   (c) gastrointestinal symptoms—dysphagia, diarrhoea (malabsorption), liver disease symptoms (uncommon);
   (d) renal tract symptoms—haematuria, hypertension, renal failure;
   (e) respiratory symptoms—symptoms of pulmonary fibrosis, pleurisy;
   (f) cardiac symptoms—symptoms of pericarditis, palpitations (arrhythmias), symptoms of cardiac failure (dilated cardiomyopathy).
2. History of exposure to silicone implants, polyvinyl chloride, L-tryptophan (eosinophilic myalgia syndrome), Spanish toxic oil, drugs (e.g., bleomycin, pentazocine). Also ask about drugs likely to aggravate Raynaud's phenomenon, e.g., beta-blockers.

3. Treatment received, e.g., D-penicillamine and side effects thereof.
4. Degree of disability, e.g., function at home, ability to work, financial security, etc.

## The Examination (Figure 3)

Make a general inspection for weight loss (due to malabsorption or dysphagia).

Look at the hands (p. 200). Look for the signs of CREST (a more benign form of scleroderma usually with oesophageal involvement causing dysphagia). Other signs are calcinosis (calcific deposits in subcutaneous tissue at the ends of the fingers), Raynaud's phenomenon (resulting in loss of tissue pulp at the ends of the fingers), sclero-dactyly (tightening of the skin on the fingers), and telangiectasia.

Inspect the nail folds using a hand-held magnifying glass for dilated capillary loops; the fourth digit is the best one to study. Note any polyarthropathy and fixed flexion deformity. Assess hand function (p. 000).

Look at the arms for skin changes and assess proximal weakness (myositis).

Examine the head. Note any alopecia. Look at the face for 'salt and pepper' pigmentation, loss of eyebrows and loss of wrinkling, 'bird-like' facies, and te-langiectasia. Check for any difficulty in closing the eyes, for dryness of the eyes (Sjögren's syndrome) and pale conjunctivae (anaemia). Check for any difficulty opening the mouth wide and for dryness and puckering of the mouth.

Look at the chest for the 'Roman breast plate' effect. Examine the cardiovascular system (p. 135) for cor pulmonale (which is the commonest cardiac manifestation), pericarditis, arrhythmias and cardiac failure. Examine the respiratory system (p. 160) for pulmonary fibrosis, reflux pneumonitis, infection, alveolar cell carcinoma and vasculitis.

Check for dysphagia (this can be done by asking the patient directly or by asking him or her to drink a glass of water whilst you listen for its entry into the stomach—this time may be greater than 10 seconds in scleroderma and CREST). Examine the abdomen for hepatosplenomegaly (p. 165) as primary biliary cirrhosis (PBC) may occasionally be associated with CREST syndrome or SLE.

Look at the legs for vasculitis and ulceration.

The blood pressure must be taken. Also check the urine analysis and temperature charts.

## Investigations

The ESR may be raised. Anaemia may be present, due to chronic disease, iron deficiency (secondary to bleeding from oesophagitis), folate or $B_{12}$ deficiency (secondary to malabsorption), or a microangiopathic haemolytic anaemia, which is usually associated with renal disease. Hypergammaglobulinaemia (particularly IgG) is present in 50% of cases. Rheumatoid factor is present in 25% and antinuclear antibody is found in 40% of cases. Anticentromere antibody is particularly associated with CREST (70%) (Table 6-33). Investigations for malabsorption and dysphagia may be necessary. Assess visceral involvement with chest X-ray films, respiratory function tests, etc.

**Figure 3.**   *Systemic Sclerosis*

GENERAL APPEARANCE
  'Bird-like' facies
  Weight loss (malabsorption)

HEAD
  Alopecia
  Eyes
    loss of eyebrows, anaemia,
    dryness (Sjögren's),
    difficulty with closing
  Mouth
    dryness, puckered
    difficulty with opening
  Pigmentation
  Telangiectasia

HANDS
  CREST—Calcinosis, atrophy
    distal tissue pulp (Raynaud's),
    sclerodactyly, telangiectasia
  Dilated capillary loops
  Small joint arthropathy and tendon
    crepitus
  Fixed flexion deformity
  Hand function

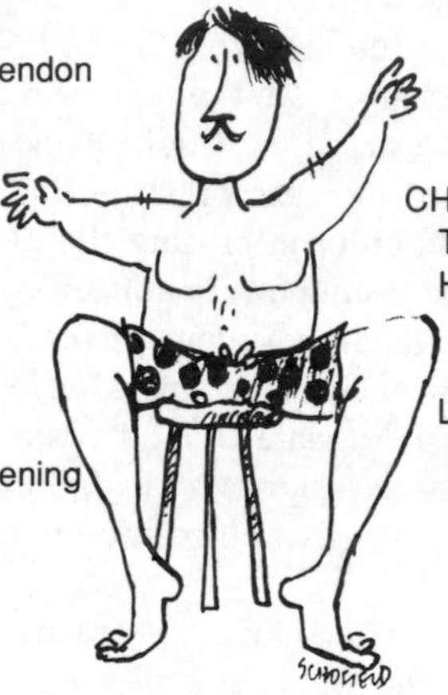

CHEST
  Tight skin ('Roman Breast Plate')
  Heart—cor pulmonale, pericardial
    effusion, pericarditis, failure,
    arrhythmias
  Lungs—fibrosis, reflux pneumonitis,
    chest infections, alveolar cell
    carcinoma, vasculitis

ARMS
  Oedema (early) or skin thickening
    and tightening
  Pigmentation
  Vitiligo
  Hair loss
  Proximal myopathy

DYSPHAGIA
  Ask patient

LEGS
  Skin lesions
  Vasculitis
  Small joint arthropathy
  Patellar crepitus

ABDOMEN
  Liver (PBC)
  Spleen

OTHER
  Blood pressure (hypertension
    in renal involvement)
  Urine analysis (proteinuria)
  Temperature chart (infection)
  Stool examination (steatorrhoea)

## Treatment

Symptomatic treatment includes avoiding vasospasm (by avoiding smoking, beta-blockers, cold weather) and treating malabsorption (particularly bacterial overgrowth, with antibiotics) and reflux oesophagitis (with $H_2$ antagonists or omeprazole). Nifedipine, phenoxybenzamine, prazosin or methyldopa may help Raynaud's phenomenon.

D-penicillamine may be helpful for skin disease and may improve survival. Pericarditis, inflammatory myopathy and early interstitial lung disease may respond to steroids.

Aggressive treatment of hypertension to delay renal failure is vital—angiotensin-converting enzyme inhibitors are the drug class of choice.

Prognosis is worse in males and those with renal or late-onset disease. Skin and gut involvement without other organ disease has the best prognosis.

# PAGET'S DISEASE

This is a disease usually of the elderly but may occur in younger patients and is characterized by excessive resorption of bone and increased formation of new bone in an irregular 'mosaic' pattern. The aetiology is unknown but may be due to a slow virus infection of osteoclasts. It presents as a management problem.

## The History

Ask about:

1. Symptoms which lead to the diagnosis:
   (a) bone pain or osteoarthritis;
   (b) change in height or hat size;
   (c) bone deformity or pathological fracture;
   (d) neurological symptoms, e.g., hearing loss, spinal cord compression, cranial nerve symptoms, headache;
   (e) symptoms of cardiac failure;
   (f) symptoms of renal colic (as there is an increased incidence of renal stones in this disease);
   (g) sarcoma of bone (rare—less than 1% of cases);
   (h) symptoms of hypercalcaemia, e.g., thirst, polyuria, nausea, coma (a rare occurrence and usually in immobilized patients or alternatively due to unrelated primary hyperparathyroidism).
2. Treatment, its effectiveness and side effects.
3. Disability at home and work.

## The Examination (Figure 4)

Inspect generally for short stature and obvious deformity.

Look at the face. Measure the skull diameter (greater than 55cm is usually

**Figure 4.**   *Paget's disease*

GENERAL INSPECTION
   Short stature
   Limb deformity
   Obvious osteosarcoma (bony swelling)

FACE
   Skull diameter (measure)
   Auscultate skull (bruits)
   Fundi-angioid streaks, optic atrophy
   Hearing (ossicle or VIII nerve
     involvement)
   Other cranial nerves (foramina
     overgrowth or platybasia)

NECK
   Short neck (platybasia)
   Jugular venous pressure—
     cardiac failure (high output)

BACK
   Deformity
   Tenderness
   Warmth
   Bruits

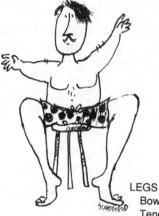

LEGS
   Bowing femur, tibia
   Tenderness, warmth, swelling bones
   Hip examination (movements)
   Knee examination

GAIT

NEUROLOGICAL ASSESSMENT OF LIMBS
   (spinal cord compression, platybasia)

OTHER
   Urine (blood)
   Height (measure)

abnormal). Look for prominent skull veins, feel for bony warmth and auscultate for systolic bruits or bronchial breath sounds. Examine the fundi for angioid streaks (p. 196) and for retinitis pigmentosa or optic atrophy which are rare. Also assess visual acuity and visual fields. Test to see if hearing is decreased due to ossicle involvement or eighth nerve compression. Remember ALL the other cranial nerves (p. 205) may rarely be affected owing to overgrowth of foramina or platybasia.

Look at the neck for platybasia. These patients have a short neck and low hairline, the head is held in extension and neck movements are decreased. Assess the jugular venous pressure and examine the heart for signs of cardiac failure due to a hyperdynamic circulation (p. 135).

Examine the back (p. 204). Note any deformity, especially kyphosis. Tap for tenderness. Feel for warmth. Auscultate for systolic bruits over the vertebral bodies.

Look at the legs for anterior bowing of the tibia and lateral bowing of the femur. Feel for warmth. Note any changes of osteoarthritis in the hips and knees. Be careful as the bones may be tender. There may be limitation of hip movements—especially abduction—and fixed flexion deformity of the knees (p. 203).

Sarcomas should be looked for, particularly in the femur, humerus and skull, usually presenting as a tender localized swelling.

A full neurological examination is necessary for spinal cord compression and platybasia in which quadraparesis may be present. If the patient is mobile, don't forget to assess walking for any disability (p. 245). Cerebellar signs may also rarely occur with platybasia.

Check the urine analysis (for blood as renal stone incidence is increased) and measure the patient's height (for serial follow-up).

## Investigations

These are indicated in symptomatic patients requiring treatment and in asymptomatic subjects to determine the extent of skeletal involvement. Routine testing for hypercalcaemia may be worthwhile, especially for any patient who is immobilized.

The serum alkaline phosphatase level is an indicator of disease activity, as is the urinary hydroxyproline level. Bone scanning is more sensitive than an X-ray film in assessing the extent of disease. Radiologically the bones most often involved are the pelvis, femur, skull and tibia. Look for bony enlargement, increased density, an irregular widened cortex and cortical infractions (incomplete pseudofractures) on the convex side of the bowed long bones. The early lytic phase of the disease presenting with a flame-shaped osteolytic wedge advancing along the bones, is often overlooked. Secondary arthritic changes may occur (e.g., hips).

## Differential Diagnosis

Paget's disease may occasionally be confused with osteoblastic bone secondaries (e.g., from prostate, Hodgkin's disease) or fibrous dysplasia.

## Treatment

The indications for treatment are bone pain, progressive deformity or complications such as neural compression or high-output cardiac failure. Non-steroidal anti-inflammatory drugs should be used first to control pain. Orthopaedic procedures such as total hip replacement may be indicated. Steroids are effective only in high doses and are therefore not recommended.

A number of drugs are available which reduce bone resorption. Calcitonin of salmon or human origin, given subcutaneously, often improves bone pain and neurological symptoms and is the drug of choice. Resistance to salmon calcitonin after 1 to 2 years may indicate the development of neutralizing antibodies. Serum alkaline phosphatase levels and urinary hydroxyproline levels are a good guide to the effect of treatment; a 50% reduction in either test value indicates a good response to treatment.

Disodium etidronate, a bisphosphonate given orally, is usually effective at reducing hydroxyproline excretion and often relieves symptoms, but may exacerbate bone pain initially. It also impairs bone mineralization and may cause osteomalacia. Newer bisphosphonates are more potent inhibitors of bone resorption and have very prolonged effects.

Mithramycin, given intravenously, can be very effective. It is reserved for occasions when rapid remission is required, e.g., spinal cord compression. There may be significant increases in bone lysis and predisposition to fractures with this drug, as well as bone marrow depression.

The appearance of sarcoma is associated with a very poor prognosis. Surgical excision is rarely curative. Little other treatment is available.

# DIABETES MELLITUS

This is a very common subject for the long case, as diabetic patients are always available. It presents usually a management, rather than a diagnostic, problem. The examiners like this disease because it tests very practical management skills. Don't forget the criteria for diagnosis of diabetes mellitus—a fasting (overnight) blood sugar level of 7.8mmol/L or higher on at least 2 separate occasions, or in the absence of fasting hyperglycaemia, a 2-hour postprandial glucose level of 11.1 mmol/L or higher.

## The History

Ask about:

1. The age at which diabetes was diagnosed and its manner of presentation, e.g., thirst, polyuria and polydipsia, weight loss, infection, ketoacidosis, asymptomatic glycosuria. Remember the rare causes of glucose intolerance (Table 6-34).

**Table 6-34.**   *Causes of Glucose Intolerance*
_____

1. Diabetes mellitus

2. Counter-regulatory hormone excess (rare)
   Acromegaly (p. 192)
   Cushing's syndrome (p. 190)
   Phaeochromocytoma
   Glucagonoma (associated with necrolytic erythema)

3. Pregnancy

4. Drugs
   Steroids or the contraceptive pill
   Streptozotocin
   Thiazide diuretics (temporary and mild, secondary to hypokalemia)
   Phenytoin, diazoxide (insulin secretion inhibited)

5. Pancreatic disease
   Chronic pancreatitis or carcinoma
   Haemochromatosis (p. 77)

6. Syndromes
   Lipoatrophic diabetes (generalized lipoatrophy, hepatomegaly, hirsutism, hyper-
   pigmentation, hyperlipidaemia)
   Type A syndrome (usually young females with acanthosis nigricans and polycystic ovary
       disease)
   Type B syndrome (acanthosis nigricans and autoimmune disease)
_____


2. The treatment initiated at diagnosis.
3. The diet prescribed. Ask what constitutes the diet. Inquire about the number of calories or portions. 1 portion = 75g of carbohydrate = 60 calories = 250 kilojoules (N.B. This definition of a portion does vary).
4. Insulin treatment. Ask about how much and when taken. Also ask where the insulin is injected and by whom.
5. The progress of the disease:
   (a) Assessment of control adequacy. Ask whether the patient tests the urine or uses a glucometer. Inquire how often the tests are done, the usual results, at what time of day the test is performed and whether the dose is adjusted at other times, c.g., gastrointestinal upset, etc.
   N.B. Symptoms of poor control:
       (i)  hyperglycaemia—polyuria, thirst, weight loss, intermittent blurring of vision, hospital admissions with ketoacidosis;
       (ii) hypoglycaemia—morning headaches, night sweats, weight gain, seizures. Ask about the time of day in relationship to food, alcohol, exercise and insulin injection.
   (b) Involvement of other systems:
       (i)  cardiovascular system, e.g., ischaemic heart disease, intermittent claudication;
       (ii) respiratory, e.g., tuberculosis;

      (iii) nervous system, e.g., peripheral neuropathy, autonomic neuropathy (causing impotence, fainting, nocturnal diarrhoea) (Table 8-37), cerebrovascular disease, amyotrophy;

      (iv) eyes, e.g., regular visits to an ophthalmologist and treatment received (especially ask about laser treatment);

      (v) renal system, e.g., dysuria, nocturia, oedema, hypertension;

      (vi) skin, e.g., boils, vaginitis (monilia), necrobiosis lipoidica (p. 199).

6. Family history of diabetes and obstetric history (e.g., big babies, stillbirths).

7. Drug history, e.g., steroids, thiazides, the contraceptive pill, beta-blockers.

8. Associated other diseases, e.g., history of pancreatitis, Cushing's syndrome (p. 190), acromegaly (p. 192).

9. Social background, e.g., type of work, living conditions (living alone or with family, etc.), coping with giving insulin (associated blindness, etc.), eating habits, financial situation.

## The Examination (p. 197)

Detailed examination is essential.

## Management

The general aim is to regulate diet, exercise and insulin so as to allow the patient to lead a normal life while avoiding short and long term complications.

### The newly diagnosed diabetic

The major management decision here is whether insulin is required. This will in some cases be obvious—e.g., for the young patient with ketoacidosis—but for many elderly, obese diabetics the position is not so clear. If insulin is not indicated at presentation, attempt to gain control first by weight loss, diet and possibly oral hypoglycaemic agents.

1. Weight loss to ideal body weight increases insulin sensitivity.

2. Realize that there is some disagreement about the ideal diet, but achieving ideal weight is essential. It is worthwhile recommending an even distribution of carbohydrate—e.g., for an average-sized patient, three portions for each meal and two portions for morning and afternoon tea and supper. A diet should contain 50% carbohydrate, and the remaining 50% should contain about half each of fat and protein. (There is some controversy about the exact proportions of fat and protein.) The diet should include high-fibre foods and poly-unsaturated fats.

3. The use of oral hypoglycaemic agents is controversial. Some endocrinologists will never use oral hypoglycaemic agents and believe that failure of weight loss and diet indicates the need for insulin. Others, however, are prepared to use them for elderly patients. There are two types of oral hypoglycaemic agents: sulphonylureas and biguanides.

    (a) Sulphonylureas include first generation drugs (e.g., glibenclamide, chlorpropamide and tolbutamide) and second generation drugs (e.g., glipizide, glypuride). Second generation drugs are as effective as the first generation and are associated with fewer drug interactions. Side effects of sulphonylureas include:

(i)     possibly an increase in cardiovascular death rate;

(ii)    prolonged hypoglycaemia;

(iii)   weight gain (due to increase in appetite);

(iv)    bone marrow depression;

(v)     cholestatic jaundice;

(vi)    skin rash;

(vii)   alcohol intolerance causing flushing (chlorpropamide only);

(viii)  water retention and hyponatraemia (chlorpropamide only).

The effectiveness of the sulphonylureas is variable.

Primary failure occurs in 40% of cases, and secondary failure in 3% to 30%; only 20% to 30% of patients continue with satisfactory control.

The mechanism of action of sulphonylureas is to increase insulin action peripherally, and to increase insulin secretion.

(b) Metformin is the only available biguanide. Side effects of biguanides include:

(i)    lactic acidosis;

(ii)   vitamin $B_{12}$ malabsorption;

(iii)  diarrhoea.

For these reasons metformin is very rarely indicated.

### Insulin Therapy

1. Insulin requirements initially are approximately half a unit per kilogram per day. Regimens include (i) split-mixed combinations of intermediate-acting insulin (e.g., monotard, NPH) and regular; (ii) Ultralente to provide a basal insulin level during the day, regular insulin before each meal or snack and intermediate insulin at bedtime; or (iii) continuous subcutaneous administration of regular insulin by an open loop infusion pump. Human insulin has replaced the highly purified (monocomponent) insulins. Aim for euglycaemia; ideally the glucose level should be between 3.5 and 7.0mmol/L throughout the day and night.

2. Insulin resistance is defined as a requirement of more than 200 units per day. Causes of insulin resistance are:

   (a) obesity (decreased receptor number);

   (b) insulin antibodies (uncommon, and an indication for a more purified insulin);

   (c) circulating antagonist hormones, e.g., growth hormone (e.g., in puberty), cortisol, thyroxine, glucagon;

   (d) association with acanthosis nigricans (Table 6-34), (e.g., receptor abnormalities, lipodystrophies). Remember injecting into a lipoatrophied site may cause poor control because of unpredictable absorption.

3. Insulin allergy causes immediate local reactions (e.g., pruritus, local pain) or delayed reactions (e.g., swelling). Urticaria and anaphylaxis can also occur. Treatment in mild cases is with antihistamines and local steroids, but in severe cases desensitization is important. Insulin allergy is more common in patients who stop and start insulin therapy.

4. The Somogyi effect is rebound morning hyperglycaemia following nocturnal hypoglycaemia, due to release of counterregulatory hormones. The treatment is to reduce the evening insulin dose. The 'dawn' phenomenon is early morning hyperglycaemia in the *absence* of nocturnal hypoglycaemia; here the treatment is to increase the insulin coverage without inducing hypoglycaemia.
5. Causes of hypoglycaemia in a previously stable diabetic on insulin therapy are:
    (a) decreased food intake, increased exercise or weight loss;
    (b) injection errors;
    (c) diabetic renal disease;
    (d) rare causes, e.g., high level of insulin antibodies, malabsorption, intestinal hurry, hypothyroidism, autoimmune adrenal insufficiency, panhypopituitarism or an insulinoma.
6. Haemoglobin A1C gives some indication of control over the preceding 3 months, but the numbers may be distorted by one or two high blood sugar levels.

### Diabetic Education

As diabetes is a lifelong disease, detailed education by the team looking after the patient is important. Regular follow-up is essential. Blood glucose monitoring with a glucometer by younger intelligent patients is very desirable—initially testing several times a day before and after meals and before bed may be necessary, but later, in stable diabetes twice daily is enough. Exercise promotes glucose utilization; in the well-controlled diabetic it is important to reduce the dose of regular insulin before exercise or supplement with glucose (NOTE: exercise in the poorly controlled diabetic may precipitate ketoacidosis because of increased release of counter-regulatory hormones).

### Management of Chronic Complications

Absolute proof that tight control prevents or reverses complications is not available. However, most clinicians agree that rigorous control is desirable.

Complications are probably due to damage caused by glycosylated proteins. Referral to an ophthalmologist is desirable if on follow-up you find diabetic retinopathy (Table 8-37, p. 200) or the duration of diabetes is greater than 5 to 10 years. Remember to control other risk factors, e.g., hypertension (for eye disease and arterial disease), smoking (for retinopathy and vascular disease) and alcohol intake (for neuropathy).

Diabetic nephropathy is a common cause of chronic renal failure and results from arteriolar disease and/or glomerulosclerosis (classical Kimmelstiel-Wilson lesion or more commonly diffuse intercapillary glomerulosclerosis). There is an increased incidence of papillary necrosis with urinary tract infection. The best form of management for end-stage chronic renal failure in a diabetic is peritoneal dialysis and early renal transplantation. Remember that diabetics with chronic renal failure invariably also have retinopathy, which may be worsened by haemodialysis.

For those with severe systemic complications or end-stage renal disease, whole-organ pancreas (with or without kidney) transplantation is a promising therapeutic option.

## The Pregnant Diabetic

Remember that blood sugar levels are normally lower in pregnancy. A woman with no diabetic history should be screened for gestational diabetes in the 24th to 28th week. A positive result for diabetes in pregnancy is a blood sugar level of 5mmol/L or higher (fasting) and 8mmol/L or higher (2 hours after a meal) on 2 occasions.

Insulin requirements vary during pregnancy owing to the effects of human placental lactogen (HPL). In the first trimester insulin requirements usually remain unchanged, but in the second trimester some increase in insulin requirements occurs owing to increasing HPL levels. By the third trimester insulin requirements are usually at least 50% higher than before pregnancy, but postpartum there is a dramatic decrease in insulin requirement.

The complications of poor control seen in the infant are:

(a) congenital malformations, e.g., spina bifida;
(b) macrosomia;
(c) intrauterine fetal deaths;
(d) immature babies, e.g., with respiratory distress syndrome, hypoglycaemia, hypocalcaemia, jaundice.

In addition to routine insulin treatment, very strict control (with use of a glucometer) is essential. It is common to admit the mother to hospital in the third trimester.

# CHRONIC RENAL FAILURE

Chronic renal failure is not a particularly common subject for the long case. However, it is a difficult and important one. The patient will usually know he or she has renal disease. Methodical questioning to establish the diagnosis, cause, management and complications is usually necessary.

## The History

### Questions Regarding Diagnosis and Aetiology

1. Glomerulonephritis (Tables 6-35 and 6-36). Determine if there is a history of proteinuria, haematuria, oliguria, oedema, sore throat, sepsis, rash, haemoptysis or renal biopsy. Ascertain treatment details, e.g., antihypertensives, immunosuppressives, antiplatelet therapy, dialysis, etc.
2. Analgesic nephropathy. Ask about the number and type of analgesics consumed, urinary tract infections, hypertension, haematuria, gastrointestinal blood loss, nocturia, renal colic (sloughed papillae, stones), transitional cell cancer and anaemia.
3. Polycystic kidneys (Table 8-17, p. 179). Ask about family history, how the disease was diagnosed, haematuria, polyuria, loin pain, hypertension, renal calculi, headache, subarachnoid haemorrhages and visual disturbance (intracranial aneurysm).

**Table 6-35.**   *The Nephrotic Syndrome*

**Clinical Features:**
1. Proteinuria (>3.5g/24h)
2. Hypoalbuminaemia (serum albumin <30g/L)
3. Oedema
4. Hyperlipidaemia (increased LDL and cholesterol)

**Causes:**
1. Primary (80%)
   Idiopathic membranous glomerulonephropathy is the commonest cause in adults over 40 years of age. Other primary causes include focal glomerulosclerosis, membranoproliferative glomerulonephritis and minimal change nephropathy.

2. Secondary
   Systemic disease, e.g., systemic lupus erythematosus (p. 97), diabetes mellitus (p. 108), Hodgkin's disease (minimal change) (p. 87), solid tumours (membranous).

   Infection, e.g., hepatitis B, HIV (focal sclerosis), infective endocarditis (p. 33), quartan malaria

   Drugs, e.g., gold, penicillamine, probenecid, high-dose captopril, non-steroidal anti-inflammatory drugs, heroin

N.B. Renal vein thrombosis is a complication and rarely a cause of the nephrotic syndrome.

**Table 6-36.**   *Classification of Glomerulonephritis*

**Primary**
*Diffuse:*
1. Minimal change
2. Membranous
3. Proliferative
   Post-streptococcal (and other post-infections)
   Mesangiocapillary
   Crescentic
   Mesangioproliferative

*Focal:*
1. IgA nephropathy
2. Focal glomerulosclerosis

**Glomerulonephritis as Part of a Systemic Disease, e.g.,**
1. Systemic Lupus Erythematosus (SLE) (p. 97)
2. Henoch-Schonlein Purpura
3. Polyarteritis Nodosa (PAN)
4. Goodpasture's Syndrome
5. Wegener's Granulomatosis
6. Infective endocarditis (p. 33)
7. Cryoglobulinaemia
8. Myeloma (p. 90)

**Table 6-37.**  *Dialysis*

| **Peritoneal Dialysis (CAPD, CCPD, or IPD)** | |
| --- | --- |
| Advantages: | Simple, reliable and safe (from a cardiovascular point of view). Removes large fluid volumes. Allows greater freedom of diet and fluid intake. Preferable for diabetics. |
| Disadvantages: | Infection. Protein loss (up to 100g/day). Basal atelectasis. Abdominal hernias. Does not control uraemia in hypercatabolic patients. Hyperglycaemia. Catheter displacement. 'Peritoneal membrane failure'. Perforation of bladder and bowel (rare). Hydrothorax (rare). |
| **Haemodialysis** | |
| Advantages: | Takes approximately 18 hours per week. No protein loss. Large volumes can be ultrafiltrated. |
| Disadvantages: | Circulatory access problems (thrombosis, infection of vascular access). Heparin may increase bleeding. Increased cardiovascular instability. Hepatitis B or C, HIV infection. Osteodystrophy. Dialysis dementia (aluminium). |

N.B. Mortality from dialysis is due to myocardial infarction (60%) or sepsis (20%) in most cases. Acquired cystic disease in native kidneys may occur; <5% are malignant. Arthropathy and carpal tunnel syndrome may occur in dialysis patients due to amyloid ($\beta_2$ microglobulin deposition)

HIV = human immunodeficiency virus; CAPD = chronic ambulatory peritoneal dialysis; CCPD = cycling chronic peritoneal dialysis (exchanges done at night); IPD = intermittent peritoneal dialysis.

4. Reflux nephropathy. Ask about childhood renal infections, cystoscopy, operations, treatment (e.g., regular antibiotics) and enuresis.
5. Diabetic nephropathy (p. 112).
6. Hypertensive nephropathy. Ask how the disease was diagnosed, duration and control of hypertension, treatment and compliance with medication, angiography, family history and any history of pregnancy-induced hypertension.
7. Connective tissue disease (especially systemic lupus erythematosus p. 97 and scleroderma, p. 102).

Ask when these were diagnosed and how they are being treated. The progression to end-stage renal disease may be rapid or very prolonged and this needs to be documented.

## Questions Regarding Management

1. Conservative management. Ask about follow-up, medications, diet, salt and water allowance, investigations performed (particularly renal biopsy), effect on the quality of life and whether erythropoietin has been given intravenously in an attempt to normalize the haematocrit.
2. Dialysis (Table 6-37). Ask about haemodialysis or peritoneal dialysis, including where performed, how often, how many hours per week, relief of symptoms with treatment and subsequent complications. Also ask about shunts, other operations (e.g., renal tract operations, parathyroidectomy) and medications taken.

3. Transplant management. Ask when and how many, whether living relative or cadaver, postoperative course, improvement, symptoms since transplantation, medications, follow-up and long-term complications (e.g., neoplasia, steroid complications) (p. 119).
4. Social arrangements. Ask about employment, the family's ability to cope, travel, sexual function and financial situation.

### Questions Regarding Complications

1. Conservatively treated patients. Ask about symptoms of anaemia, bone disease, secondary gout or pseudogout, pericarditis, hypertension, cardiac failure, peripheral neuropathy, pruritus, peptic ulcers and impaired cognitive function.
2. Dialysis patients. Ask about shunt blockage, infection, etc.
3. Transplant patients. For patients with recent transplants ask about graft pain or swelling (failure of graft function, rejection), infection, urine leaks, steroid side effects. For those with long-term renal grafts, ask about serum creatinine, proteinuria, recurrent glomerulonephritis, avascular necrosis, skin cancer, and reflux nephropathy (p. 119).

## The Examination (Figure 5)

A complete physical examination is always essential. Look particularly for the following.

1. General appearance. Mental state, hyperventilation, Kussmaul's breathing, hiccuping and the state of hydration.
2. Hands. Nails: Terry's nail in chronic renal failure ('half and half nails'—a distal brown arc at least 1mm wide may be seen in one-third of cases but is also seen in 2% of normal subjects); brown lines near the ends of the nail (Muehrcke's lines) in nephrotic syndrome; Mee's lines (transverse white bands) in arsenic poisoning. Also, palm crease pallor, vasculitis, vascular shunts at the wrist, asterixis, peripheral neuropathy.
3. Arms. Bruising, pigmentation, scratch marks, subcutaneous calcification, myopathy, fistulae.
4. Face. Eyes for jaundice, anaemia and band keratopathy (due to hypercalcaemia); mouth (dry, fetor); rash (e.g., SLE).
5. Chest. Pericardial rub, cardiac failure, lung infection, pleural effusion, venous hum (shunt).
6. Abdomen (p. 179). Costovertebral angle tenderness (push with the thumb), palpable kidney, scars (due to dialysis or transplants), renal artery bruit (a continuous bruit or systolic-diastolic bruit in the upper abdomen suggests significant renal artery stenosis), bladder area, rectal examination (for prostatomegaly, urethral mass and signs of blood loss), nodes (lymphoma, cytomegalovirus or other infections if the patient is immunosuppressed), ascites (dialysis or other causes), femoral bruits and pulses.
7. Urine for blood, protein, specific gravity, pH, glucose and urine microscopy.
8. Legs. Oedema, bruising, pigmentation, scratch marks, peripheral neuropathy, vascular access (for shunts), myopathy.

**Figure 5.** *Chronic Renal Failure*

GENERAL INSPECTION
Mental state
Hyperventilation (acidosis), hiccups
Sallow complexion
Hydration

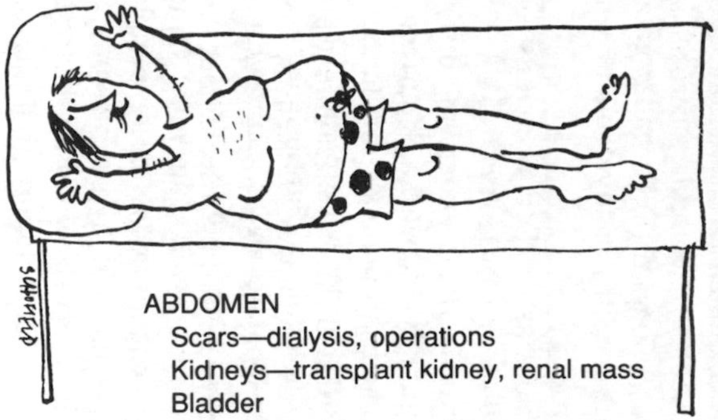

ARMS
Bruising
Pigmentation
Scratch marks
Urea frost (whole crystal deposits—terminal uraemia)
Myopathy

FACE
Eyes—anaemia, jaundice, band keratopathy
Mouth—dryness, fetor
Rash (vasculitis, etc.)

HANDS
Nails—Terry's nails, brown lines
Vascular shunts
Asterixis
Neuropathy

ABDOMEN
Scars—dialysis, operations
Kidneys—transplant kidney, renal mass
Bladder
Liver
Lymph nodes
Ascites
Bruits
Rectal (prostatomegaly, bleeding)

OTHER
Blood pressure—lying and standing
Fundoscopy—hypertensive and diabetic changes, etc.

CHEST
Heart—pericarditis, failure
Lungs—infection

LEGS
Oedema—nephrotic syndrome, cardiac failure, etc.
Bruising
Pigmentation
Scratch marks
Gout
Neuropathy
Vascular access

BACK
Tenderness
Oedema

URINE ANALYSIS
Specific gravity, pH
Glucose—diabetes
Blood—'nephritis', infection, stone, etc.
Protein—'nephritis', etc.

SCHOFIELD

9. Back. Bone tenderness, sacral oedema.
10. Blood pressure and pulse lying and standing. Fundoscopy (p. 209).

## Investigations

1. Determine renal function.
   (a) Glomerular filtration rate—24-hour creatinine clearance and plasma creatinine/urea level.
   (b) Tubular function—plasma electrolyte levels, urine specific gravity and pH, glycosuria, serum phosphate and uric acid, aminoaciduria.
   (c) Urine analysis and 24-hour urinary protein excretion.
   (d) Other if necessary, e.g., [131]I-hippurate scan to help determine the potential for return of renal function in obstructive uropathy, gallium scan.
2. Determine renal structure.
   (a) Plain X-ray film of the abdomen (KUB—kidneys, ureters, bladder).
   (b) Ultrasound.
   (c) High-dose intravenous pyelogram (IVP) under good hydration (but avoid in patients with diabetes mellitus or myeloma or when the creatinine level is >150µmol/L).
   (d) CT scan (same restrictions as for IVP if contrast is to be used).
   (e) Cystoscopy and retrograde pyelography.
3. Investigations aimed towards the likely underlying disease process, e.g., measurement of antinuclear antibody, hepatitis B surface antigen, complement, immune complexes, immunoelectrophoresis, micturating cystogram, etc.
4. Investigations aimed at assessing the widespread effects of renal failure, e.g., blood count, serum ferritin level, midstream urine examination, calcium, phosphate and alkaline phosphatase levels, parathyroid hormone level, nerve conduction studies, arterial Doppler studies, etc.
5. The following all favour chronic over acute renal failure: nocturia, polyuria, long-standing hypertension, renal osteodystrophy, peripheral neuropathy, anaemia, severe hyperphosphataemia and hyperuricaemia. The differentiation of acute and chronic renal failure is also aided by determining kidney size; they are usually small in chronic renal failure, but the exceptions to this rule include:
   (a) diabetic nephropathy (early);
   (b) polycystic kidneys;
   (c) obstructive uropathy;
   (d) acute renal vein thrombosis;
   (e) amyloidosis;
   (f) rarely other infiltrative diseases, e.g., lymphoma (pp. 87–90), which can all produce chronic renal failure but maintain normal kidney size.

In general, however, kidneys enlarge or maintain normal size in acute renal failure and are small in chronic renal failure.

Always ask about previous urine analyses, e.g., insurance examinations in which proteinuria may have been detected and followed up, giving a clue about chronic glomerulonephritis.

Lastly, anaemia and burr cells in the peripheral blood film are usually evidence of chronic renal failure, but may occur in acute renal failure, e.g., in systemic lupus erythematosus (p. 97), thrombotic thrombocytopenic purpura, haemolytic uraemic syndrome.

## Treatment

Normally this is a very long-term problem (see Table 6-38).

1. Treat reversible causes of detrioration. There include:
    (a) hypertension
    (b) urinary tract infection;
    (c) urinary tract obstruction;
    (d) dehydration;
    (e) cardiac failure;
    (f) drug use, e.g., radiocontrast (especially in diabetes, myeloma), non-steroidal anti-inflammatory drugs, aminoglycosides;
    (g) hypercalcaemia;
    (h) hyperuricaemia with urate obstruction;
    (i) ·hypothyroidism or rarely hypoadrenalism.
2. Monitor and control the blood pressure very carefully.
3. Carefully attend to salt and water balance and acidosis.
4. Watch the calcium and phosphate levels (Table 6-38).
5. Restrict dietary protein.
6. Dialyse when indicated.
7. Consider transplantation.

The indications for dialysis (Table 6-37) are:

1. Uraemic symptoms despite conservative management.
2. Volume overload despite salt and water restriction and diuretic use.
3. Hyperkalaemia unresponsive to conservative measures.
4. Progressive deterioration of renal function (dialyse before symptoms develop).
5. Dialyse early in acute renal failure.

# RENAL TRANSPLANTATION

Renal transplantation is now a widely accepted, commonly performed treatment for end-stage renal failure. Patients unfortunately continue to have a number of chronic problems which may bring them into hospital and make them available for examinations. Cadaveric transplantation is much more common in this country than the use of matched family donors. The prognosis continues to improve and the introduction of cyclosporin has made a big difference to survival rates in both groups of patients. One-year survival is now over 80% in experienced centres. Contraindications to renal transplant include malignancy, an untreatable focus of infection and severe extrarenal disease.

**Table 6-38.** *Complications and Treatment of Chronic Renal Failure*

**Anaemia**
Causes include: erythropoietin deficiency, poor nutrition (especially folate deficiency), blood loss, haemolysis, bone marrow depression, chronic disease and aluminium toxicity.

Treatment should include prophylactic folate supplements for dialysis patients. Iron is rarely required. Erythropoietin is very effective for the chronic anaemia of renal failure and can normalize the haematocrit; it is particularly useful for the transfusion-dependent patient. Transfusion should be undertaken only for very severe unresponsive anaemia or in preparation for transplantation.

**Bone Disease**
Maintenance of normal calcium and phosphate levels is the key to preventing the problem. Treatment with calcium supplements, vitamin D analogues and phosphate-binding resins is necessary.

1. Osteomalacia. Diagnosis by:
   a) X-ray films (decreased density, Looser's zones)
   b) low calcium, phosphate and vitamin D levels
   c) high serum alkaline phosphatase level
   d) bone biopsy (tetracycline labelled)
2. Secondary Hyperparathyroidism. Diagnosis by:
   a) X-ray film (microcysts on radial side of the middle phalanx, erosion of the clavicular ends, 'Rugger jersey' spine, telescoped terminal phalanges, metastatic calcification of vessels)
   b) high phosphate and parathyroid hormone levels, but a normal calcium level
   c) bone biposy (tetracycline labelled)
3. Osteoporosis
4. Osteosclerosis

**Peripheral Neuropathy**
The treatment of this is peritoneal dialysis/transplantation.

**Hypertension**
This needs careful monitoring and control.

**Infection**
This is due to both the disease and the drugs given to treat glomerulonephritis.

**Acidosis**
This should be treated with sodium bicarbonate or dialysis and carefully monitored.

**Hyperkalaemia**
This should be treated with a low potassium diet and ion-exchanging resins if necessary. Dialysis is very effective.

# The History

1. Ask the patient about the cause of the original renal failure (p. 113). Find out how long the transplant has been in situ and whether this is the first transplant. Ask whether the kidney came from a relative or was a cadaveric graft.
2. Ask the patient if blood transfusions were received before the renal graft. In the pre-cyclosporin era, patients who had never had a blood transfusion had a 20% to 30% increased incidence of graft failure, but this is much less with the use

of cyclosporin. Probably more than 5 units of blood are required for optimal effect.

3. The patient should be well informed about previous rejection episodes and how these have been managed. Find out whether this is the reason for the current admission. Clinically rejection may be marked by fever and swelling and tenderness over the graft. There is also often a reduction in urine volume. The patient should be aware of all these signs. Ask about recent graft biopsies which may have been necessary to assess rejection or disease recurrence.
4. Find out what immunosuppressive drugs the patient is taking and in what doses. He or she should know whether changes in doses have been required recently because of any problems with any of the drugs.
5. Ask about specific complications of immunosuppression. Cyclosporin can result in significant side effects (p. 79). Ask about ischaemic heart disease and peripheral vascular disease since the incidence of these conditions remains higher in these patients than in the general population.

## The Examination

Look particularly at the skin for squamous and basal cell carcinomas. Note any signs of Cushing's syndrome (p. 190). Examine the abdomen carefully, noting the position and site of the allograft and whether it has any tenderness or bruits. Look for old vascular access sites for haemodialysis and decide whether there will be problems finding sites for access for further dialysis if this is required.

Examine the lungs for signs of infection and the mouth for candida. Look at the temperature chart.

## Investigations

1. It is important to obtain the serum creatinine level as well as the creatinine clearance rate and if possible establish whether the creatinine level has been rising or falling since the time of the transplant. A slightly elevated creatinine level is considered acceptable in patients on cyclosporin treatment since this drug interferes with renal function.
2. The electrolyte levels and liver function test results are important. Cyclosporin can cause hepatotoxicity (p. 79).
3. A white cell count should be obtained to look for leukocytosis (infection or steroids) and leukopenia (e.g., excessive doses of azathioprine). The azathioprine dose is usually adjusted according to the neutrophil count. The haemoglobin usually rises towards normal levels in patients with a successful transplant.
4. The results of blood cultures should be sought if there has been any suggestion of recent infection. Urinary tract infection must also be considered and early urine microscopy is helpful.

## Management

Probably the majority of patients receiving chronic dialysis are candidates for renal transplantation. The donor's kidneys should be ABO compatible. Typing by

HLA DR antigens may improve graft survival. Immediately after transplantation management problems include acute tubular necrosis, infection, cyclosporin nephrotoxicity and rejection episodes. Rejection is prevented with the use of steroids, azathioprine and cyclosporin. Acute rejection episodes are treated with three pulse doses of 0.5 to 1g of intravenous methylprednisolone or anti-OKT3. Azathioprine is given in doses of 1.5 to 3mg/kg/day; it is metabolized by the liver so its dose does not need to be varied according to renal function, but the dose is usually adjusted according to the neutrophil count. Prednisone is given in maintenance doses of approximately 10mg daily after about 6 months. A gradually rising creatinine may be a sign of cyclosporin toxicity or of chronic rejection. This is a difficult clinical problem, but graft biopsy can often be used to decide whether the cyclosporin should be stopped or immunosuppression should be increased.

The major cause of graft loss is chronic rejection. Recurrence of glomerulonephritis in the transplanted kidney occasionally occurs and is most common with focal glomerulosclerosis; IgA nephropathy, Goodpasture's syndrome and membranoproliferative glomerulonephritis (especially type II) can also recur.

# MULTIPLE SCLEROSIS

This is a common chronic disease. Patients suffering from multiple sclerosis are easily available for the examinations. They are mostly very well informed about, and interested in, their disease. Multiple sclerosis usually begins in early adult life and is commoner in females.

## The History

Diagnosis requires at least two neurological events separated in time and place within the central nervous system. Multiple sclerosis is primarily a clinical diagnosis.

1. Presenting symptoms (listed in approximate order of importance):
    (a) episodes of spastic paraparesis, hemiparesis, or tetraparesis (may present as gradually progressive disease in late onset multiple sclerosis);
    (b) episodes of limb paraesthesia (due to posterior column, medial lemniscus or internal capsule involvement);
    (c) episodes of visual disturbance—loss of acuity, pain on eye movement, loss of central visual field (optic neuritis);
    (d) episodes of ataxia (due to cerebellar or posterior column involvement);
    (e) band sensations around trunk or limbs;
    (f) less common symptoms, e.g., vertigo, symptoms of cranial nerve disorders (e.g., tic douloureux), urinary urgency, incontinence of faeces, impotence, depression, euphoria, dementia, seizures, bulbar dysfunction (pseudobulbar palsy).
2. Ask about precipitating factors, e.g., heat (hot baths, etc.), infection, fever, pregnancy and exercise.
3. Ask about family history (multiple sclerosis is 8 times more common in

immediate relatives and occurs more frequently in subjects with HLA B7 and DW2 and less frequently in subjects with HLA B12).

4. Ask about social disability, e.g., sexual function, work, financial problems.
5. Ask about place of birth (multiple sclerosis is 10 times more common in subjects who spent their childhood in temperate latitudes than in tropical regions).

## The Examination

The signs may be very variable. Look particularly for signs of spastic paraparesis and posterior column sensory loss (p. 239) as well as cerebellar signs (p. 245).

Examine the cranial nerves (p. 205). Look carefully for loss of visual acuity, optic atrophy, papillitis, and scotomata (usually central). Internuclear ophthalmoplegia is an important sign and is almost diagnostic in a young adult. It can also occur in patients with systemic lupus erythematosus or Sjögren's syndrome who may have disease confined to the central nervous system, or with brainstem tumours or infarcts. Internuclear ophthalmoplegia is weakness of adduction in one eye due to damage of the medial longitudinal fasciculus; there may be nystagmus in the abducting eye. In multiple sclerosis internuclear ophthalmoplegia is often bilateral. Other cranial nerves can be affected (III, IV, V, VI, VII, pseudobulbar palsy). Charcot's triad consists of nystagmus, intention tremor and scanning speech, but occurs in only 10% of patients.

Look for Lhermitte's sign (which is an electric shock-like sensation in the limbs or trunk following neck flexion). This can also be caused by other disorders of the cervical spine such as subacute combined degeneration of the cord, cervical spondylosis, cervical cord tumour, foramen magnum tumours and mantle irradiation.

Rarely Devic's disease, usually seen in children, may be present (bilateral optic neuritis and transverse myelitis occurring within a few weeks of one another) and may be a variant of multiple sclerosis.

## Differential Diagnosis

The differential diagnosis of multiple central nervous system lesions includes systemic lupus erythematosus (p. 97), Sjögren's syndrome, polyarteritis nodosa, Behçet's disease, acute disseminated encephalomyelitis, subacute myelo-optic neuritis, meningovascular syphilis, paraneoplastic effects of carcinoma, sarcoidosis (p. 58), Lyme disease, and multiple emboli from any source.

It is important to distinguish multiple sclerosis affecting predominantly the spinal cord from other diseases—especially subacute combined degeneration of the cord (commoner in the older population) (p. 241) and spinal cord compression presenting with root pain and persistent sensory levels (p. 239).

## Investigations

Multiple sclerosis is essentially a clinical diagnosis, but the following tests may be helpful.

1. Cerebrospinal fluid in chronic multiple sclerosis contains oligoclonal IgG bands (70%) and an altered IgG-albumin ratio. Myelin basic protein may be elevated in acute demyelination. There are usually fewer than 50 white cells per millilitre in the cerebrospinal fluid, but acute severe demyelination may result in a cell count exceeding 100/mL.
2. CT scan may reveal low-density sometimes contrast enchancing plaques in white matter (subcortical or paraventricular, but only in 10% to 50% of cases). Magnetic resonance imaging (MRI) is the imaging modality of choice but may be negative in up to 10% of patients with definite multiple sclerosis.
3. Visual evoked responses are delayed in 80% of established cases and indicate past optic neuritis (important if there is only one other clinically detectable lesion present). Other helpful tests are auditory evoked responses and somatosensory evoked responses which may indicate lesions elsewhere in the white matter. However, evoked potentials are less reliable than studies on cerebrospinal fluid and magnetic resonance imaging.

## Treatment

General support is essential. During exacerbations bed rest with meticulous nursing is vital. Treatment of bladder dysfunction, severe spasticity (e.g., with baclofen), tic douloureux and facial spasm (e.g., carbamazepine and physiotherapy) is important.

ACTH or corticosteroids given during acute exacerbations may lessen the severity of symptoms and speed recovery. The final extent of disability is not affected, however. Cyclophosphamide and steroids are used for chronic progressive disease, but this is not universally accepted treatment since side effects may outweigh any benefit.

Copolymer I (a polymer of myelin basic protein) has been reported to reduce the frequency of exacerbations when used at an early stage of disease. Alpha and beta interferon may also help, but gamma interferon causes neurological deterioration.

# MYASTHENIA GRAVIS

This disease presents both diagnostic and management problems. Peak incidence in females is in the third decade, but in males it is in the seventh decade. Overall it is more common in females (2:1).

## The History

Ask about:

1. Symptoms at presentation:
   (a) ocular—diplopia (90%), drooping eyelids;
   (b) bulbar—choking (weakness of pharyngeal muscles), dysarthria, trouble chewing;

   (c) limb girdle—proximal muscle weakness, there is fatigue on exertion and
       prompt partial recovery on resting.
2. History of difficult anaesthesia (due to prolonged weakness after muscle relaxation) and past episodes of pneumonia (due to bulbar and respiratory weakness).
3. How the diagnosis was made, including whether an edrophonium test was
   performed.
4. History of thymectomy.
5. Other treatment—including drug dose and when the last dose was taken, plasma
   exchange.
6. Drug use may interfere with neuromuscular transmission (p. 126).
7. Other organ-specific autoimmune disease associations (p. 195).
8. Social history.

## The Examination

Examine for muscle fatigue, particularly the oculomotor muscles (tested by sustained upward gaze), bulbar muscles (tested by counting or reading aloud) and the
proximal limb girdles (tested by holding the arms above the head). Weakness of
neck flexion may be prominent. Reflexes are preserved. There is no sensory loss.
Muscle atrophy is usually minimal. Look for a thymectomy scar.

## Investigations

Tests for myasthenia gravis include:

1. The Tensilon test—edrophonium is given intravenously and if muscle strength
   improves dramatically, myasthenia gravis is likely.
2. Acetylcholine receptor antibodies. These occur in 80% to 90% of cases with
   false-positive results being rare (but the frequency is lower in pure ocular and
   inactive myasthenia gravis). The titre is not directly related to disease severity.
   Antistriated muscle antibody is detectable in 90% of patients with thymoma but
   is also common in elderly patients without a thymoma.
3. Electromyogram (EMG). In myasthenia gravis repetitive stimulation at low fre-
   quencies causes a progressive reduction in muscle action potential amplitudes
   if that particular muscle is affected.
4. Thymoma investigations, e.g., chest X-ray film, thoracic CT scan.

## Treatment

### Symptomatic
Anticholinesterases are the mainstay of treatment in mild cases. Pyridostigmine is
the usual one given. Potassium supplements and potassium-sparing diuretics (e.g.,
spironolactone) may give additional improvement.

### Disease-suppressing
Steroids are indicated for generalized severe disease when anticholinesterases are
inadequate. They are then needed in the long term. They may aggravate disease

initially (in the first week to 10 days), so all patients should be in hospital when treatment is commenced. Failed steroid treatment in patients with severe disease is an indication for immunosuppressive drug therapy (e.g., azathioprine, cyclosporin).

Thymectomy is advisable early for every patient with generalized myasthenia gravis. Thymomas occur in 10% of cases (and of these 25% are malignant) and thymic hyperplasia occurs in 65%. Of such patients, after resection, 70% show improvement and 25% undergo remission. Causes of failed response to thymectomy include incomplete removal, ectopic tissue and fulminant disease.

Plasmaphaeresis is useful in acute situations such as in myaesthenic crisis, preparation for surgery or in the peripartum period.

Prognosis of myasthenia gravis is good; 50% of patients have a remission, although 5% to 10% die from respiratory failure.

It is important to avoid drugs which interfere with neuromuscular transmission, like streptomycin, gentamicin, quinidine and procainamide.

## Differential Diagnosis

The differential diagnosis of proximal muscle weakness is important (p. 243).

The Eaton-Lambert syndrome may occasionally be confused with myasthenia gravis. This syndrome results from presynaptic failure of release of acetylcholine, caused by small cell carcinoma of the lung (in 50% of cases) or autoimmune disease. There is proximal muscle weakness and pain, and power may increase on repeated effort. Reflexes are reduced or absent. The ocular and bulbar muscles are usually spared. The EMG is helpful (high-frequency stimulation causes an increment, while low-frequency stimulation causes a decrement). Symptoms may be reduced by guanidine or 3, 4 diaminopyridine, and the underlying tumour is managed appropriately; steroids and plasma exchange therapy can also be effective.

# GUILLAIN–BARRÉ SYNDROME

*All CN except I II, VIII*

This disease is not uncommon in the examination as patients may be in hospital for an extended period and present management difficulties. It is the most common acute polyneuropathy and it can affect both sexes and all ages.

## The History

Ask about:

1. The presenting symptoms of ascending motor weakness, their time course, and whether decreasing or increasing. The patient may report difficulty breathing. Other symptoms include paraesthesiae or sensory loss (sensory neuropathy is usually minimal) and symptoms of cranial nerve palsies, particularly bulbar lesions (all cranial nerves except I, II and VIII can be affected).
2. Preceding respiratory or gastrointestinal infection (which occurs in 50% of

cases 1 to 3 weeks before). Other precipitating events, e.g., surgical operation, vaccination, intercurrent malignant disease (e.g., Hodgkin's disease) (p. 87) and systemic lupus erythematosus (p. 97) should be enquired about.

3. Previous episodes of disease (in chronic relapsing polyneuropathy).
4. Symptoms of autonomic neuropathy, e.g., postural hypotension, difficult to control arrhythmias (Table 8-37).
5. Social history.

## The Examination (p. 226)

Predominantly distal muscle weakness without atrophy is present, although 25% have more proximal than distal weakness. The upper limbs may be more affected than the lower limbs. Muscle tenderness is common (one-third of cases). Signs of autonomic neuropathy must be looked for. Sensory loss is usually minimal, but if present affects the posterior columns (vibration and proprioception) more than the spinothalamic tracts. Always measure forced expiratory time (p. 160). Look for a urinary catheter.

## Differential Diagnosis

Infectious mononucleosis, acute viral hepatitis or mycoplasma pneumonia can cause the Guillain-Barré syndrome. The differential diagnosis of acute ascending motor paralysis includes diphtheria, polio, polyarteritis nodosa, acute intermittent porphyria, tick or snake bites and rhabdomyolysis.

The differential diagnosis of autonomic neuropathy includes diabetes mellitus (p. 199), alcoholism, acute intermittent porphyria and amyloidosis.

## Investigations

Guillain-Barré syndrome is a clinical diagnosis. Helpful tests include:

1. Excluding the above-mentioned causes, e.g., by Monospot test, cold agglutinins.
2. Cerebrospinal fluid examination. Look for a raised protein level (increased gammaglobulin) and lack of cells in 90% of cases; 10% have 10 to 50 mononuclear cells per high-power field.
3. Respiratory function tests ($FEV_1$, FVC) to assess progressive involvement of respiratory muscles; the patients can progress rapidly (even over hours) to respiratory failure.
4. Nerve conduction and electromyogram (EMG) studies. Many nerves may have to be studied to find abnormalities because this disease is patchy. Abnormalities include slowed motor conduction, conduction blocks, increased distal motor latencies, reduced sensory action potentials and increased F wave latencies. EMG evidence of denervation takes 10 days to 3 weeks to appear and indicates axonal involvement with a worse prognosis.

## Treatment

Physiotherapy to prevent contractures is important. Respiratory support in an intensive care unit is essential if the vital capacity is less than 800mL.

Steroids (and ACTH) are not beneficial. Plasmaphaeresis shortens the time to recovery from respiratory paralysis and hastens the return of mobility.

Prognosis is good—most patients make a complete recovery but 2% die (usually of respiratory complications, pulmonary emboli, cardiac arrhythmia) and 10% have a major residual deficit. If the deficit does not diminish in 3 weeks or the patient has autonomic neuropathy, a poorer prognosis is more likely.

# PYREXIA OF UNKNOWN ORIGIN (PUO)

While not a common long case, this problem presents both diagnostic and management problems. The term 'pyrexia of unknown origin' is used only for patients with a fever >38.3°C (101°F) for ≥3 weeks where no diagnosis has been made during a week of intensive study. The common causes are listed in Table 6-39.

## The History

Ask about:

1. Chronological development of symptoms. Gastrointestinal tract symptoms should be sought (e.g., subphrenic abscess, diverticular abscess, cholangitis, appendiceal abscess, liver abscess, Crohn's disease, metastatic cancer in the abdomen, Whipple's disease). Note any preceding acute infections, e.g., diarrhoeal illness, boils. Chest pain may suggest pericarditis, multiple pulmonary emboli or rarely intraluminal dissection of the aorta. Joint pain may suggest rheumatoid arthritis, systemic lupus erythematosus, vasculitis, atrial myxoma or endocarditis. Dysuria or rectal pain may indicate prostatic abscess or urinary tract infection. Headache and joint or muscle pain may indicate giant cell arteritis. Night sweats may indicate lymphoma, tuberculosis, brucellosis, endocarditis or an abscess.
2. Places of residence and overseas travel (e.g., malaria, amoebiasis, fungal infections).
3. Contact with domestic or wild animals or birds, (e.g., psittacosis, brucellosis, Q fever, histoplasmosis, leptospirosis, toxoplasmosis).
4. Close contact with persons who have tuberculosis.
5. Occupation and hobbies, e.g., veterinary surgeon, farming (fungal infection, raw milk ingestion, hypersensitivity pneumonitis).
6. Sexual practices (e.g., risk of HIV infection, venereal disease, pelvic inflammatory disease).
7. Evidence of immunocompromised host, e.g., cytomegalovirus, pneumocystis.

**Table 6-39.** *Important Causes of Pyrexia of Unknown Origin*

1. Neoplasms
   a) Lymphoma, leukaemia, malignant histiocytosis
   b) Solid tumors
      Primary—renal, lung, atrial myxoma, large bowel, pancreas, liver
      Secondary—metastatic disease (including melanoma, sarcoma)
2. Infections
   a) Bacterial—tuberculosis, atypical mycobacteria, abscess (e.g., pelvic, abdominal),
      brucellosis, endocarditis, pericarditis, osteomyelitis, cholangitis, pyelonephritis,
      leptospirosis
   b) Viral, rickettsial and chlamydial—hepatitis, HIV, cytomegalovirus, Q fever, psittacosis
   c) Parasitic—malaria, amoebiasis, trichinosis, toxoplasmosis.
3. Connective tissue diseases
   a) Rheumatoid arthritis, systemic lupus, rheumatic fever, adult Still's disease
   b) Vasculitis, e.g., polyarteritis nodosa, temporal arteritis, Wegener's granulomatosis
4. Miscellaneous
   a) Drug fever
   b) Inflammatory bowel disease, Whipple's disease
   c) Granulomatous disease, e.g., granulomatous hepatitis, sarcoid (uncommon)
   d) Multiple pulmonary emboli, intraluminal aortic dissection
   e) Thyroiditis
   f) Haematomas, e.g., retroperitoneal space (consider especially if on anticoagulants)
   g) Haemolysis
   h) Habitual hyperthermia (usually young females with low-grade fever but no organic
      disease)
   i) Thermoregulatory disorders (rare—abnormal temperature regulating mechanism)
   j) Cyclic neutropenia
   k) Factitious fever

8. Medication used, e.g., drug fever (antibiotic allergy, sulphonamides, bromides, arsenicals, iodides, thiouracils, barbiturates, laxatives—especially those containing phenolphthalein).
9. Anticoagulant use (accumulation of old blood in a closed space, e.g., retroperitoneal, perisplenic).
10. Iatrogenic infection, e.g., catheter, arteriovenous fistula, prosthetic heart valve.
11. Factitious fever from injection of contaminated material or tampering with thermometer readings. Suspect the former diagnosis if there is an excessively high temperature, or the latter in the absence of tachycardia, chills or sweats.

## The Examination

Look at the temperature chart if available to see if the fever pattern is characteristic. The temperature tends to fall to normal each day in pyogenic infections, tuberculosis and lymphoma, while in malaria the temperature can return to normal for days before rising again. Inspect the patient; note if he or she appears ill or not, if there is cachexia (suggesting a chronic disease process) and any skin rash (e.g., erythema multiforme, erythema nodosum).

Pick up the hands and look for stigmata of infective endocarditis, any vasculitic changes and for finger clubbing. Inspect the arms for injection sites (intravenous drug abuse). Palpate for epitrochlear and axillary lymphadenopathy (e.g., lymphoma, solid tumor spread, focal infections).

Examine the eyes for iritis or conjunctivitis (e.g., connective tissue disease, sarcoid) or jaundice (e.g., cholangitis, liver abscess). Look in the fundi for choroidal tubercles (miliary tuberculosis), Roth's spots (infective endocarditis), retinal haemorrhages or infiltrates (e.g., leukaemia). Note any facial rash (e.g., systemic lupus erythematosus). Feel the temporal arteries (temporal arteritis). Examine the mouth for ulcers, gum disease, and the teeth and tonsils for infection. Feel the parotids for parotitis and the sinuses for sinusitis. Palpate the cervical lymph nodes. Also examine for thyroid enlargement and tenderness (subacute thyroiditis).

Examine the chest. Palpate for bony tenderness over the sternum and shoulders. Carefully examine the respiratory system (e.g., for signs of tuberculosis, abscess, empyema, carcinoma) and the heart for murmurs (e.g., infective endocarditis, atrial myxoma) or prosthetic heart sounds or rubs (e.g., pericarditis).

Examine the abdomen. Inspect for skin rash (e.g., rose-coloured spots of typhoid). Palpate for tenderness (e.g., abscess), hepatomegaly (e.g., granulomatous hepatitis, hepatoma, cirrhosis, metastatic deposits), splenomegaly (e.g., haemopoietic malignancy, infective endocarditis, malaria), renal enlargement (e.g., obstruction, renal cell carcinoma). Feel the testes for enlargement (e.g., seminoma, tuberculosis). Feel for inguinal adenopathy.

Always ask for the results of the rectal examination (e.g., prostatic abscess, rectal cancer, Crohn's disease) and pelvic examination (pelvic pus). Look at the penis and scrotum for a discharge or rash.

Finally examine the nervous system for signs of meningism (chronic meningitis) or focal neurological signs (e.g., brain abscess, mononeuritis multiplex in polyarteritis nodosa). Check the results of urine analysis.

## Investigations

Determine how many blood cultures have been obtained and the results. Ask to review the blood count and smear (e.g., for neutropenia, eosinophilia, atypical lymphocytes, etc.), liver function tests, electrolytes and creatinine. Look at the chest X-ray. If urinary tract disease is suspected, an intravenous pyelogram is important. Selected serologies may be helpful depending on the clinical setting (e.g., fungal, HIV, Q fever). Check the PPD for tuberculosis exposure and an anergy panel. If abdominal disease is suspected or other tests have not provided a clue, obtain an abdominal ultrasound and/or CT scan.

Biopsy of involved tissue (e.g., bone marrow, liver, lymph node, skin, muscle) may lead to a definitive diagnosis. The clinical setting determines what should be biopsied.

Exploratory laparotomy when all other tests are negative and in the absence of any evidence of abdominal disease is usually unproductive.

# Treatment

Therapy directed at the underlying disease should be the goal of assessment. Therapeutic trials in the absence of a diagnosis (e.g., antibiotics, antituberculosis therapy, non-steroidal anti-inflammatory drugs, steroids) may result in resistant bacterial infection or drug toxicity, and may impair making an accurate diagnosis.

# Chapter 7

# THE SHORT CASE

*You see, but you do not observe.*

Sir Arthur Conan Doyle (1859–1930)

This is a test of ability to examine a patient smoothly, confidently and accurately. There is rarely the opportunity to go back and repeat the examination. It takes a long time to get used to being watched critically whilst examining. This is why it is important to have done short cases of every conceivable type so that the physical examination is performed automatically the correct way. Whilst proceeding the candidate should be consciously synthesizing the results, not trying to remember what to do next.

Listen carefully to the introduction given. The examiner will often give a hint, so be attentive. Usually a short history will be given (e.g., this patient presented with chest pain) to indicate the problem, followed by an instruction to examine a particular system or organ (e.g., the cardiovascular system). These specific instructions must be followed. For example, if asked to examine a patient's gait, it is vital to get the patient to walk first. This may appear obvious, but many candidates have failed because they have not followed their examiner's instructions. Time is a major factor here—it is limited and one does not want to run out of time before having got to the problem the examiner has raised.

There is no official time limit for each short case, but candidates are expected to do at least 2 cases in 22 minutes. We suggest people aim to examine each short case proficiently within 7 minutes. The commonest short cases are cardiovascular and neurological problems. Abdominal examinations are probably next in importance. There has been more emphasis on rheumatological assessment in recent years.

It is a good idea, when introduced to the patient, to step over and shake his or her hand firmly. This may endear one to the patient (and exclude dystrophia myotonica) (p. 244). Always position the patient properly (e.g., at 45 degrees for the cardiovascular examination or flat for the abdominal examination) and make sure the appropriate parts are undressed.

Do not ask the patient any questions, with few exceptions. It is prudent to say

'Let me know if I hurt you', and, when examining the abdomen directly, ask 'Are you tender anywhere?' This is a test of bedside manner (and may give you a clue!). Always try to make the patient comfortable and avoid totally exposing him or her, or exposing parts not being examined.

It is always worthwhile taking a moment to stand back and look at the whole patient. This may well prevent one missing an obvious 'spot' diagnosis, e.g., myxoedema, a thymectomy scar in a patient with muscle weakness (myasthenia), a psoriatic rash in a patient with arthropathy, or a Cushingoid appearance in a hypertension examination. Practice really does help improve the ability to see clinical associations. A candidate will almost always fail if a major sign is missed.

Do remember that the candidate is in fact demonstrating the signs (particularly in the case of a neurological short case) to the examiners. It is important to perform each manoeuvre accurately and deliberately. Be seen to be smooth and confident, as if the examination has been done a thousand times before. Also try to be confident of each sign before moving on to another area, e.g., on finding an abdominal mass, concentrate on excluding the various possibilities and coming to a firm conclusion and don't primarily worry about the time it takes. Practice will facilitate formation of conclusions accurately and quickly.

The examiners may pull a candidate away in the middle of the examination. This is why it is important to be synthesizing the data as one goes. Do not get flustered—this usually means enough of the examination has been completed for you to have discovered the important signs. It is at this stage that the examiners may require the interpretation of a particular sign in isolation (e.g., the collapsing carotid pulse in aortic incompetence or the double apex beat in hypertrophic cardiomyopathy).

More often, there is no interruption until the examination is almost finished. We suggest the candidate just keep on examining until told to stop and then list all the other things he or she would like to have done (e.g., urine analysis, rectal examination).

Before presenting the findings, listen closely to the examiner's instruction. A candidate will often be asked 'What did you find?', when he or she will be expected to describe the relevant signs first and then comment on possible causes. Sometimes candidates may be asked 'What is your diagnosis?', when they will be expected to give a diagnosis or differential diagnosis first and then list the signs which support the contention.

One useful method of presentation is to first repeat the examiner's introduction, then give the findings, e.g., 'I was asked to examine Mr Jones, a 60-year-old man who presented with dyspnoea. On examination of his cardiovascular system, Sir, I found....' When describing the signs it is probably easiest to present them in the order that they were looked for, e.g., for the cardiovascular system, pulse rate then blood pressure, jugular venous pressure, etc. It is important to state all the positive signs and the important negative ones. Be definite about each sign mentioned or do not mention the sign at all. There is no place for expressions like 'slightly asymmetrical,' 'minor', 'early clubbing', etc. Never use the phrase 'I think'; it will always be interpreted as uncertainty.

Confidence is critical to success in the short cases. Do not lose confidence if an error is made, just continue on—the examiner may not even have noticed. If the examiner detects hyperventilation, tremor or other signs of extreme anxiety, he or she may well wonder, perhaps unfairly, if the candidate is capable of handling other stresses, e.g., during a cardiac arrest.

A short differential diagnosis is usually expected even if the diagnosis is obvious, e.g., a patient with fasciculation, plus upper and lower motor neurone signs in the legs and no sensory loss, almost certainly has motor neurone disease, but a non-metastatic manifestation of carcinoma must be considered. Always mention common before rare diseases, and always consider the patient's age and gender. Never reel off any old list; the differential diagnosis must be tailored to the particular patient seen.

After presentation of the signs, usually 3 minutes or more are set aside for discussion. Sometimes a chest X-ray film or ECG (if relevant) will be shown to the candidate. Usually management and therapeutic aspects are not discussed in the short case.

The College is attempting to move away from the traditional 'spot' short case (e.g., acromegaly) and concentrate more on 'realistic' cases, e.g., heart murmurs, abdominal masses. However, all types still crop up—the candidate must try to prepare for most possibilities.

There are 2 golden rules to remember:

1. Do EVERYTHING properly when you examine—NEVER take short cuts.
2. Don't say ANYTHING wrong when presenting—it is better to say you don't know.

# Chapter 8
# COMMON SHORT CASES

*The trouble with doctors is not that they don't know enough,*
*but that they don't see enough.*

Corrigan (1802–1880)

## INTRODUCTION

You may be asked to examine a system or a particular part of the patient, or just observe the whole patient for a 'spot' diagnosis.

In the following pages a system for examining major short case possibilities will be outlined. Use these to help develop your own system. A few useful lists are also included in this section.

In all cases, before beginning a specific examination, you should stand back for a moment and carefully observe the patient. Otherwise you may miss the associated 'spot' diagnosis, e.g., peripheral neuropathy in a myxoedematous patient or aortic incompetence in a patient with Marfan's syndrome.

The patient will normally be positioned and undressed for you. However, if either positioning or undressing is unsatisfactory, you must insist on having this corrected.

## THE CARDIOVASCULAR SYSTEM

### Cardiovascular Examination

This patient presents with dyspnoea on exertion and orthopnoea. Please examine the cardiovascular system.

### *Method* (Figure 6)
Position the patient at 45 degrees and make sure the chest and neck are fully exposed. In a female the requirements of modesty dictate you should cover her breasts with a towel or loose garment.

**Figure 6.** *Cardiovascular System*

GENERAL INSPECTION (Lying at 45°)
Marfan's, Turner's,
Down's syndrome
Rheumatological disorders,
e.g., anklosing spondylitis
(aortic incompetence)
Acromegaly, etc.
Dyspnoea

HANDS
Radial pulses—right and left
Radiofemoral delay
Clubbing
Signs of infective endocarditis—
splinter haemorrhages, Osler's
nodes, etc.
Peripheral cyanosis
Xanthomata

BLOOD PRESSURE

FACE
Eyes
Cornea: arcus cornea
Sclerae: pallor, jaundice
Pupils: Argyll Robertson
(aortic incompetence)
Xanthelasma
Malar flush (mitral stenosis,
pulmonary stenosis)
Mouth
Cyanosis
Palate (high arched—Marfan's)
Dentition

NECK
Jugular Venous Pressure
Central venous pressure height
Wave form (especially large *v* waves)
Carotids
pulse character

PRAECORDIUM
Inspect
Scars—whole chest, back
Deformity
Apex beat—position, character
Abnormal pulsations

Palpate
Apex beat
position
character
Thrills
Abnormal impulses
N.B. Beware of dextrocardia

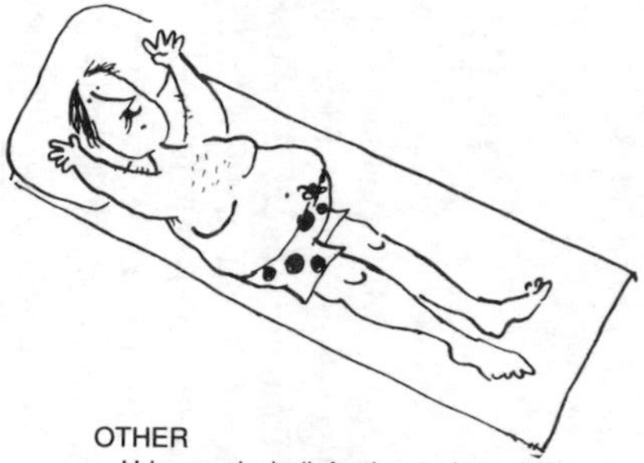

OTHER
Urine analysis (infective endocarditis)
Fundi (endocarditis)
Temperature chart (endocarditis)

Auscultate
Heart sounds
Murmurs
Position patient
left lateral position
sitting forward (forced expiratory
apnoea)
N.B. Palpate for thrills again on
positioning
Dynamic Auscultation
Respiratory phases
Valsalva
Exercise (isometric, e.g., handgrip)
Standing
Squatting

BACK (sitting forward)
Scars, deformity
Sacral oedema
Pleural effusion (percuss)
Left ventricular failure (auscultate)

ABDOMEN (Lying flat—1 pillow only)
Palpate liver (pulsatile, etc.), spleen,
aorta
Percuss for ascites (right heart failure)
Femoral arteries—palpate, auscultate

LEGS
Clubbing toes
Cyanosis, cold limbs, trophic
changes, ulceration (peripheral
vascular disease)
All peripheral pulses
Oedema
Xanthomata
Calf tenderness

**Table 8-1.**  *Jugular Venous Pulse*

---

1. Wave Form
Causes of Dominant *a* Wave:
   Tricuspid stenosis (also causes a slow *y* descent)
   Pulmonary stenosis
   Pulmonary hypertension
Causes of a Dominant *v* Wave:
   Tricuspid incompetence
Causes of Cannon *a* Waves:
   Complete heart block
   Paroxysmal nodal tachycardia with retrograde atrial conduction
   Ventricular tachycardia with retrograde atrial conduction or atrioventricular dissociation

2. Causes of an elevated central venous pressure
   1. Right ventricular failure
   2. Tricuspid stenosis or incompetence
   3. Pericardial effusion or constrictive pericarditis
   4. Superior vena caval obstruction
   5. Fluid overload
   6. Hyperdynamic circulation, e.g., fever, anaemia, thyrotoxicosis, arteriovenous fistula, pregnancy, exercise, beri beri, hypoxia, hypercapnia

---

Inspect whilst standing back for the appearance of Marfan's, Turner's or Down's syndromes. Also look for dyspnoea and cyanosis.

Pick up the patient's hand. While feeling the radial pulse, ask if you may take the blood pressure. Examiners will usually supply you with the reading. Make sure you remember this. Inspect the hands then for clubbing, and for capillary pulsations if there is a possibility of aortic incompetence. Also look for the peripheral stigmata of infective endocarditis (p. 33)—splinter haemorrhages are common (and are also caused by trauma), while Osler's nodes and Janeway lesions are rare. Look quickly, but carefully, at each nail bed, otherwise it is easy to miss these signs. Note any tendon xanthomata (type II hyperlipidaemia, p. 41).

The pulse at the wrist should be timed for rate and rhythm. Pulse character is poorly assessed here. This is also the time to feel for radiofemoral delay (which occurs in coarctation of the aorta) and radial-radial inequality.

Next inspect the face. Look at the eyes briefly for Argyll-Robertson pupils, jaundice (valve haemolysis) and xanthelasma (type II or III hyperlipidaemia). You may also notice the classical 'mitral facies' (owing to dilatation of malar capillaries associated with severe mitral stenosis because of pulmonary hypertension and a low cardiac output). Then inspect the mouth using a torch for a high-arched palate (Marfan's syndrome), petechiae and state of dentition (endocarditis). Look at the tongue or lips for central cyanosis.

The neck is very important. The jugular venous pulse (JVP) must be assessed for height and character (Table 8-1 and Figure 7). Use the right internal jugular vein to assess this. Look for a change with inspiration (Kussmaul's sign).

Now feel each carotid pulse separately (never together!). Assess the pulse character (Table 8-2).

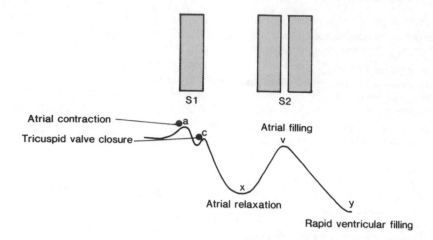

**Figure 7.**  *The jugular venous pulse, and its relationship to the first (S1) and second (S2) heart sounds.*

**Table 8-2.**  *Arterial Pulse Character*

| | |
|---|---|
| Anacrotic— | small volume, slow upstroke, plus *a* wave on the upstroke. Cause : Aortic stenosis. |
| Plateau— | slow upstroke. Cause: Aortic stenosis. |
| Bisferiens— | anacrotic plus collapsing. Cause: Aortic stenosis plus Aortic incompetence. |
| Collapsing— | Causes: Aortic incompetence, Hyperdynamic circulation (qv) Arteriosclerotic aorta (elderly patients particularly), Patent ductus arteriosus, Peripheral arteriovenous aneurysm. |
| Small Volume— | Causes: Aortic stenosis, Pericardial effusion. |
| Alternans— | alternating strong and weak beats. Cause: Left ventricular failure. |

Proceed to the praecordium. Always begin by inspecting for scars, deformity, site of the apex beat and visible pulsations. Don't forget about pacemaker boxes. Mitral valvotomy scars (under the left breast) can be quite lateral and very easily missed (with ghastly repercussions in the test).

Palpate for the apex beat position. Be seen to count down the correct number of interspaces. The normal position is the fifth intercostal space, 1cm medial to the midclavicular line. The character of the apex beat is important. There are two types. A PRESSURE-LOADED (hyperdynamic, systolic overloaded) apex beat is a forceful and sustained impulse (e.g., in aortic stenosis, hypertension). A VOLUME-LOADED (hyperkinetic, diastolic overloaded) apex beat is a forceful, but unsustained impulse (e.g., in aortic incompetence, mitral incompetence). Don't miss the tapping apex beat of mitral stenosis (a palpable first heart sound). The double or triple apical impulse in hypertrophic cardiomyopathy is very important too. Feel also for an apical thrill and time it.

Then palpate with the heel of your hand for a left parasternal impulse which indicates right ventricular hypertrophy or left atrial enlargement. Now feel at the base of the heart for a palpable pulmonary component of the second heart sound ($P_2$) and aortic thrills. Percussion is usually unnecessary.

Auscultation begins with listening in the mitral area with both the bell and the diaphragm. Listen for each component of the cardiac cycle separately. Identify the first and second heart sounds (Table 8-3) and decide if they are of normal intensity and whether they are split. Now listen for extra heart or prosthetic heart sounds (Tables 8-3 and 8-4) and for murmurs (Table 8-5). Do not be satisfied at having identified one abnormality—it is more common to get complex than simple lesions in the examination.

Repeat the approach at the left sternal edge and then the base of the heart (aortic and pulmonary areas). Time each part of the cycle with the carotid pulse. Always listen below the left clavicle for a patent ductus arteriosus murmur, which may be audible here and nowhere else.

It is now time to reposition the patient, first in the left lateral position. Again feel the apex beat for character (particularly tapping). Auscultate carefully for mitral stenosis with the bell. Next sit the patient forward and feel for thrills (with the patient in full expiration) at the left sternal edge and base. Then listen in those areas, particularly for aortic incompetence.

Dynamic auscultation should always be done if there is any doubt about the diagnosis. The Valsalva manoeuvre should be performed whenever there is a pure systolic murmur. Hypertrophic cardiomyopathy is easily missed otherwise (p. 153). The patient who seems familiar with the Valsalva manoeuvre may well have a murmur affected by it.

The patient is now sitting up. Percuss the back quickly to exclude a pleural effusion (e.g., due to left ventricular failure) and auscultate for inspiratory crackles (left ventricular failure) (p. 160). If there is radiofemoral delay, also listen for a coarctation murmur here. Feel for sacral oedema and note any back deformity (e.g., ankylosing spondylitis (p. 204) with aortic incompetence).

Next lie the patient flat and examine the abdomen properly (p. 165) for hepatomegaly (right ventricular failure) and a pulsatile liver (tricuspid incompetence). Feel for splenomegaly (endocarditis) and an aortic aneurysm. Palpate both femoral arteries and auscultate here if there is any possibility of aortic incompetence (for 'pistol shots' in systole with very severe incompetence or Duroziez's sign where a systolic and diastolic murmur is heard on lightly compressing the artery with the stethoscope). Go on and examine all the peripheral pulses. Look particularly for peripheral oedema, clubbing of the toes, Achilles tendon xanthomata, signs of peripheral vascular disease, and stigmata of infective endocarditis.

At the end ask the examiners for results of the urine analysis (haematuria in endocarditis) and a temperature chart (fever in endocarditis) and examine the fundi (for Roth's spots in endocarditis and for hypertensive changes).

It is most unlikely that you will have time to complete all aspects of your examination. You may be stopped at any time (e.g., before auscultating) and asked for an opinion. Alternatively you may be asked just to examine the praecordium

**Table 8-3.** *Heart Sounds*

**First Heart Sound (S1)**
Loud—Mitral Stenosis, Tricuspid Stenosis, Tachycardia, Hyperdynamic Circulation
Soft— Mitral Incompetence, Calcified Mitral Valve, Left Bundle Branch Block, First Degree
   Heart Block

**Second Heart Sound (S2)**
*Aortic (A2)*
Loud—Congenital aortic stenosis, Systemic hypertension
Soft— Calcified aortic valve, Aortic incompetence (when the leaflets cannot coapt)
*Pulmonary (P2)*
Loud—Pulmonary hypertension
Soft— Pulmonary stenosis
*Increased Normal Splitting (wider on inspiration)*
Right bundle branch block, Pulmonary stenosis, Ventricular septal defect, Mitral incompetence
   (earlier A2)
*Fixed Splitting*
Atrial septal defect
*Reversed Splitting (P2 first)*
Left bundle branch block, Aortic stenosis (severe), Coarctation of aorta, Patent ductus
   arteriosus (large)

**Third Heart Sound (S3)**
Mechanism: Possibly tautening of the mitral or tricuspid cusps at the end of rapid diastolic
   filling.
Causes:
*Left Ventricular Third Heart Sound (S3) (louder at apex and on expiration)*
Physiological (under 40 years of age or during pregnancy), Left ventricular failure, Aortic
   incompetence, Mitral incompetence, Ventricular septal defect, Patent ductus arteriosus
*Right Ventricular Third Sound (S3) (louder at left sternal edge and on inspiration)*
Right ventricular failure, Constrictive pericarditis

**Fourth Heart Sound (S4)**
Mechanism: A high atrial pressure wave is probably reflected back from a poorly compliant
   ventricle. It is always abnormal.
Causes:
*Left Ventricular Fourth Heart Sound*
Aortic stenosis, Acute mitral incompetence, Systemic hypertension, Ischaemic heart disease,
   Hypertrophic cardiomyopathy
*Right Ventricular Fourth Heart Sound*
Pulmonary hypertension, Pulmonary stenosis

**Table 8-4.** *Prosthetic Heart Valves: Physical Signs*

| Type | Mitral | Aortic |
|---|---|---|
| Starr-Edwards* (ball valve) | Sharp opening sound after S2; sharp closing sound at S1; 'rattles' in diastole; systolic ejection murmur | Sharp opening sound after S1; sharp closing sound at S2[1]; 'rattles' in systole; systolic ejection murmur |
| Bjork-Shiley* (tilting disc) | Soft opening sound after S2; sharp closing sound at S1; no murmur | Soft opening sound after S1; sharp closing sound at S2; systolic ejection murmur |
| Xenograft[†] | Systolic ejection murmur | Systolic ejection murmur |

* Severe prosthetic dysfunction causes absence of the opening or closing sounds. Ball and cage valves cause more haemolysis than other types, while tilting disc valves are more thrombogenic.

† Biprosthetic obstruction or patient prosthetic mismatch causes diastolic rumbling.

Modified with permission from Stein JH (ed) Internal Medicine 3rd ed, 1990: Boston: Little Brown, 1987:486.

**Table 8-5.** *Differential Diagnosis of Murmurs*

| | |
|---|---|
| Pansystolic: | Mitral incompetence (p. 143), Tricuspid incompetence (p. 147), Ventricular septal defect (p. 154), Aortopulmonary shunts |
| Midsystolic: | Aortic stenosis (p. 146), Pulmonary stenosis (p. 147), Hypertrophic cardiomyopathy (P. 153), Pulmonary flow murmur of an atrial septal defect (p. 142) |
| Early Systolic: | Ventricular septal defect (either very small, or large plus pulmonary hypertension), Acute mitral incompetence, Tricuspid incompetence |
| Late Systolic: | Mitral valve prolapse (p. 144), Papillary muscle dysfunction (e.g., hypertrophic cardiomyopathy) |
| Early Diastolic: | Aortic incompetence (p. 145), Pulmonary incompetence |
| Mid-diastolic: | Mitral stenosis (p. 142), Tricuspid stenosis, Atrial myxoma, Austin Flint murmur of aortic incompetence, Carey-Coombs murmur of acute rheumatic fever |
| Presystolic: | Mitral stenosis, Tricuspid stenosis, Atrial myxoma |
| Continuous*: | 1. Patent ductus arteriosus (p. 155) |
| | 2. Arteriovenous fistula (coronary artery, pulmonary, systemic) |
| | 3. Venous hum (situated over the right supraclavicular fossa and abolished by ipsilateral compression of the internal jugular vein) |
| | 4. Rupture of a sinus of valsalva into the right atrium or ventricle |
| | 5. Aortopulmonary connection (e.g., Blalock Shunt) |
| | 6. 'Mammary souffle' (in late pregnancy or early post-partum period) |

* Aortic stenosis and aortic incompetence or mitral stenosis and mitral incompetence may be confused with a continuous murmur.

or the heart. In this case start the examination at the praecordium, but glance at
the JVP and palpate the carotid artery when auscultating.

If you are stopped, mention the list of things you would still like to do which
are particularly relevant.

If you have auscultated and there is nothing obvious at first, consider the following and exclude them:

1. Mitral stenosis (position and exercise if necessary).
2. Atrial septal defect (p. 154) (listen carefully for fixed splitting).
3. Mitral valve prolapse (perform a Valsalva manoeuvre) (p. 144).
4. Pulmonary hypertension (qv).
5. Constrictive pericarditis (p. 147).

# Notes on Valve Diseases

After you have made a diagnosis of a valve lesion, the following are the types of
facts you should know.

## Mitral Stenosis

Valve area: Normal, 4 to 6cm$^2$. Severe mitral stenosis, less than 1cm$^2$.

Causes:

1. Rheumatic (in females more often than males).
2. Congenital rarely (e.g., parachute valve, with all chordae inserting into one
   papillary muscle).

Clinical signs of severity:

1. Small pulse pressure.
2. Early opening snap (due to increased left atrial pressure).
3. Length of the mid-diastolic rumbling murmur (persists as long as there is a
   gradient).
4. Diastolic thrill at the apex (rare).
5. Presence of *pulmonary hypertension*, the signs of which are:
   (a) prominent *a* wave in the jugular venous pressure pattern;
   (b) right ventricular impulse;
   (c) loud pulmonary component of the second heart sound ($P_2$);
   (d) pulmonary incompetence;
   (e) tricuspid incompetence.

Results of investigations:

1. Electrocardiogram (ECG):
   (a) *P* mitrale in sinus rhythm;
   (b) right axis deviation (severe disease);
   (c) right ventricular systolic overload (severe disease);
   (d) atrial fibrillation.
2. Chest X-ray film (p. 149):
   (a) Mitral valve calcification.

   (b) Big left atrium
       (i)   double left atrial shadow;
       (ii)  displaced left main bronchus;
       (iii) big left atrial appendage.
   (c) Signs of pulmonary hypertension
       (i)   large central pulmonary arteries;
       (ii)  pruned peripheral arterial tree.

   N.B. If the investigations suggest left ventricular hypertrophy is present in the presence of a mitral stenosis murmur, consider these other possibilities:

   (a) associated mitral incompetence;
   (b) associated aortic valve disease;
   (c) associated hypertension;
   (d) associated ischaemic heart disease;
   (e) the possibility of right ventricular hypertrophy (with clockwise rotation) on the ECG being confused with left ventricular hypertrophy.

Echocardiograph (M Mode 2D and Doppler)
   The posterior mitral leaflet maintains its anterior position in diastole and this is pathognomonic. A delayed mitral closure with decreased EF slope is not pathognomonic, but is very suggestive. There may be heavy echoes from thickened or calcified mitral leaflets. Mitral valve area can be quite accurately determined by two-dimensional echo and Doppler measurements.

Indications for surgery:

   If there is progressive dyspnoea, pulmonary oedema or major haemoptysis that has failed to respond to medical therapy.

## Mitral Incompetence

Causes—chronic:

1. Rheumatic (males more often than females)—rarely is mitral incompetence the only murmur present.
2. Mitral valve prolapse.
3. Papillary muscle dysfunction:
   (a) left ventricular failure;
   (b) ischaemia.
4. Connective tissue disease, e.g., rheumatoid arthritis (p. 92), ankylosing spondylitis (p. 204).
5. Congenital, e.g., parachute valve, endocardial cushion defect, corrected transposition.

Causes—acute:

1. Infective endocarditis (perforation of anterior leaflet) (p. 33).
2. Myocardial infarction (chordae rupture or papillary muscle dysfunction).
3. Surgery.
4. Trauma.

Clinical signs of severity:

1. Small-volume pulse.
2. Enlarged left ventricle.
3. Third heart sound (a very important sign).
4. Early diastolic rumble.
5. Soft first heart sound.
6. Aortic component of second heart sound is earlier.
7. Pulmonary hypertension.

Results of investigations:

1. Electrocardiogram:
   (a) *P* mitrale;
   (b) right axis deviation;
   (c) left ventricular diastolic overload;
   (d) atrial fibrillation.
2. Chest X-ray film:
   (a) large (may be gigantic) left atrium;
   (b) increased left ventricle size;
   (c) valve calcification;
   (d) pulmonary hypertension (much less common).
3. Echocardiography:
   (a) thickened leaflets—rheumatic aetiology;
   (b) prolapsing leaflets;
   (c) left atrial size;
   (d) left ventricular size and function;
   (e) Doppler detection of incompetent jet in left atrium;
   (f) other valve abnormalities.

Indications for surgery:

In chronic mitral incompetence, consider surgery if there are class III or IV symptoms (p. 40) or if there is left ventricular dysfunction. In acute mitral incompetence, operate if there is haemodynamic collapse.

## Mitral Valve Prolapse (Systolic Click-Murmur Syndrome)

This is the commonest heart lesion in the community (5% to 10% of the population) and is commoner in females.

Dynamic auscultation: The click murmur is affected by:

1. Valsalva manoeuvre (decreases preload): murmur longer.
2. Handgrip (increases afterload) or squatting (increases preload): murmur shorter.

Associations:

1. Marfan's syndrome (p. 158).
2. Atrial septal defect (secundum) in 20% of cases.
3. Hypertrophic cardiomyopathy.

Complications:

1. Mitral incompetence.
2. Infective endocarditis (rare).
3. Arrhythmias (very rare).
4. Embolism (very rare).
5. Sudden death (very rare).

## *Aortic Incompetence*

Causes of chronic aortic incompetence:
Valvular:

1. Rheumatic (rarely the only murmur in this case).
2. Congenital (e.g., bicuspid valve; ventricular septal defect—an associated prolapse of the aortic cusp is not uncommon).
3. Seronegative arthropathy, especially ankylosing spondylitis.

Aortic Root (murmur may be maximal at the right sternal border):

1. Marfan's syndrome.
2. Aortitis (e.g., seronegative arthropathies, rheumatoid arthritis, tertiary syphilis).
3. Dissecting aneurysm.
4. The elderly.

Causes of acute aortic incompetence (Note: murmur may be soft because of increased left ventricular end-diastolic pressure):

1. Valvular: infective endocarditis.
2. Aortic Root: Marfan's syndrome, hypertension, dissecting aneurysm.

Clinical signs of severity in chronic aortic incompetence:

1. Collapsing pulse.
2. Wide pulse pressure.
3. Length of the *decrescendo* diastolic murmur.
4. Third heart sound (left ventricular).
5. Soft aortic component of the second heart sound ($A_2$).
6. Austin Flint murmur.
7. Left ventricular failure.

N.B. A loud systolic murmur, rarely with a thrill, may be present without any organic aortic stenosis being associated. The peripheral signs of aortic incompetence are the clue that this is the real lesion in this situation.

Results of investigations:

1. Electrocardiogram:
   (a) left ventricular hypertrophy (diastolic overload).
2. Chest X-ray film:
   (a) left ventricular hypertrophy;
   (b) valve calcification.

3. Echocardiography:
   (a) aortic root dimensions;
   (b) valve cusp thickening or prolapse;
   (c) vegetations;
   (d) left ventricular dimensions and function;
   (e) Doppler estimation of size of regurgitant jet.

Indications for Surgery:

1. Symptoms—exertional angina, dyspnoea on exertion, syncope.
2. Worsening left ventricular function, e.g., low ejection fraction (in aortic incompetence this is increased until late, severe disease intervenes) measured on a gated blood pool scan.

## Aortic Stenosis

Valve Area: 1.5 to 2.0cm$^2$. Significant stenosis at <1cm$^2$. In critical aortic stenosis, less than 0.7cm$^2$/m$^2$ or a valve gradient greater than 6.67kPa (50mmHg).

Causes:

1. Rheumatic (rarely isolated).
2. Degenerative senile calcific aortic stenosis (commonest cause in the elderly).
3. Calcific bicuspid valve.

Clinical signs of severity:

1. Plateau pulse.
2. Aortic thrill (very important sign of severe stenosis).
3. Length and lateness of the peak of the systolic murmur.
4. Fourth heart sound.
5. Paradoxical splitting of the second heart sound (delayed left ventricular ejection and aortic valve closure).
6. Left ventricular failure (a late sign—right ventricular failure is preterminal).

Results of investigations:

1. Electrocardiogram:
   (a) left ventricular hypertrophy (systolic overload).
2. Chest X-ray film:
   (a) left ventricular hypertrophy;
   (b) valve calcification.
3. Echocardiography:
   (a) valve cusp mobility;
   (b) left ventricular hypertrophy;
   (c) Doppler estimation of gradient.

Indications for Surgery:

1. Symptoms—exertional angina, exertional dyspnoea, exertional syncope.
2. Critical obstruction (based on catheterization data) and severe left ventricular hypertrophy even if asymptomatic.

## Tricuspid Incompetence

Look for the following signs:

1. The JVP: large *v* waves; the JVP is elevated if right ventricular failure has occurred.
2. Palpation: right ventricular heave.
3. Auscultation: a pansystolic murmur maximal at the lower end of the sternum and on inspiration may be present, but the diagnosis can be made on the basis of the peripheral signs alone.
4. Abdomen: a pulsatile, large and tender liver is usually present; ascites and oedema with pleural effusions may also occur.
5. Causes of tricuspid incompetence:
   (a) functional (no disease of the valve leaflets)—right ventricular failure;
   (b) rheumatic—only very rarely does tricuspid incompetence occur alone, usually mitral valve disease is also present;
   (c) infective endocarditis (right-sided endocarditis in intravenous drug abusers);
   (d) congenital—Ebstein's anomaly;
   (e) tricuspid valve prolapse (rare);
   (f) right ventricular papillary muscle infarction;
   (g) trauma (usually a steering wheel injury to the sternum).

## Pulmonary Stenosis (in adults)

Look for the following signs:

1. General signs: peripheral cyanosis because of a low cardiac output.
2. The pulse: normal or reduced, because of a low cardiac output.
3. The JVP: giant *a* waves because of right atrial hypertrophy; the JVP may be elevated.
4. Palpation: right ventricular heave; thrill over the pulmonary area.
5. Auscultation: the murmur may be preceded by an ejection click; a harsh ejection systolic murmur maximal in the pulmonary area and on inspiration is present; S4 may be present (due to right atrial hypertrophy).
6. Abdomen: presystolic pulsation of the liver may be present.
7. Signs of severe pulmonary stenosis: an ejection systolic murmur peaking late in systole; absence of an ejection click (also absent when the pulmonary stenosis is infundibular—i.e., below the valve level); presence of S4; signs of right ventricular failure.
8. Causes of pulmonary stenosis:
   (a) congenital;
   (b) carcinoid syndrome.

## Chronic Constrictive Pericarditis

This diagnosis must not be missed. The patient may appear cachexic. Look for the following signs:

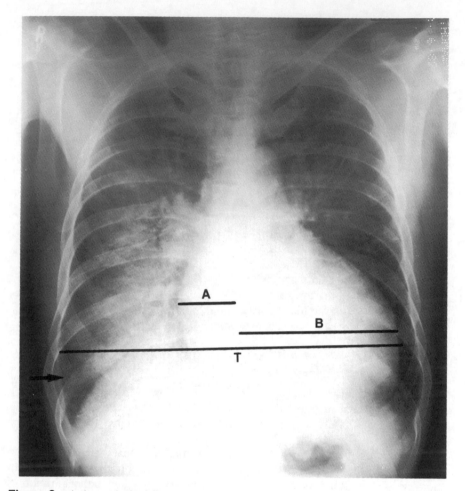

**Figure 8.** *Left ventricular failure*

- Large left ventricle (apex downwards and outwards).
  N.B. A large right ventricle causes the apex to pass upwards and outwards.
- Perihilar alveolar oedema, extending into the right lower zone.
- Small effusion tracking up the right costal margin.
- Kerley 'B' lines (oedematous interlobular septa) (arrow).
- Cardiothoracic ratio ($\frac{A+B}{T}$) is greater than the normal 50%. The thoracic measurement (T) is taken at the level of the right hemidiaphragm. The cardiac diameter is the addition of the two widths A and B.

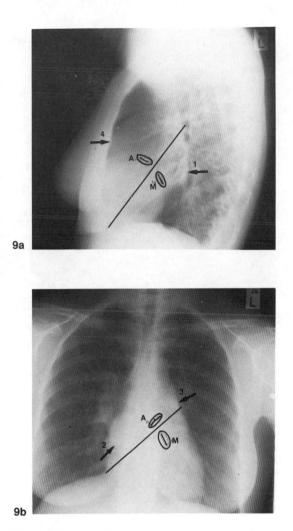

9a

9b

**Figures 9a and 9b.** *Mitral valve disease*

There is an enlarged left atrium—it enlarges posteriorly (arrow 1) and causes a double right heart border (arrow 2). The left atrial appendage also enlarges and causes a bulge below the left hilum (arrow 3).

There is secondary right ventricular enlargement (arrow 4). The right ventricle should only lie against the lower third of the anterior chest wall between the antero-inferior costophrenic recess and the manubriosternal junction.

This is an example of mitral stenosis.

*Position of the valves*

The mitral valve (M) lies below, behind, and slightly to the left of the aortic valve (A).

To distinguish the valves if calcification is present, draw imaginary lines. The PA view line passes from the right cardiophrenic angle to the inferior aspect of the left hilum. The lateral view line passes from the antero-inferior angle through to the mid-point of the hilum.

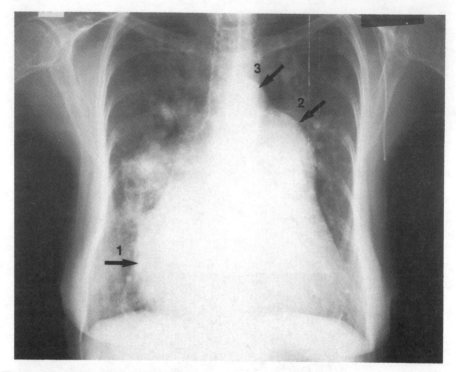

**Figure 10.** *Atrial septal defect (ASD) with Eisenmenger reaction*

- Large heart with prominent right atrium (arrow 1).
- Dilated main pulmonary artery (arrow 2) and its central branches.
- Aortic knuckle is small (arrow 3), reflecting decreased aortic flow in ASD.
- The Eisenmenger reaction shows as an abrupt narrowing of the peripheral vessels. In ordinary ASD there is pulmonary plethora.

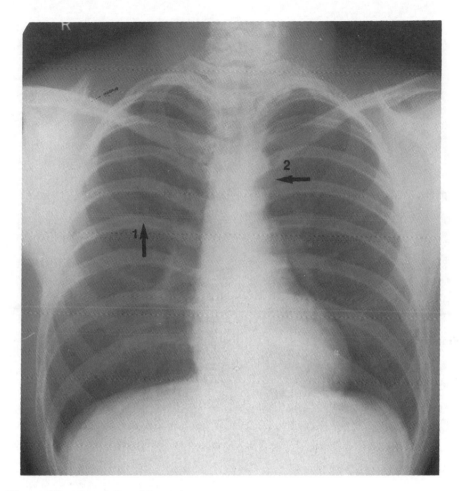

**Figure 11.** *Coarctation of the aorta*

- Lower rib notching bilaterally (arrow 1).
- Diminished aortic knuckle (arrow 2).
- This patient has not yet developed left ventricular failure.

*Differential diagnosis of inferior rib notching*
1. Coarctation of the aorta.
2. Venous obstruction (superior or inferior vena cava, innominate, or subclavian).
3. Pulmonary artery atresia.
4. Blalock-Taussig procedure (unilateral) for Fallot's tetralogy.
5. Neurofibromatosis (also causes upper rib notching).
6. Hyperparathyroidism (also causes upper rib notching).
7. Arterio-venous fistula of chest wall (intercostal artery-vein).
8. Normal variant.

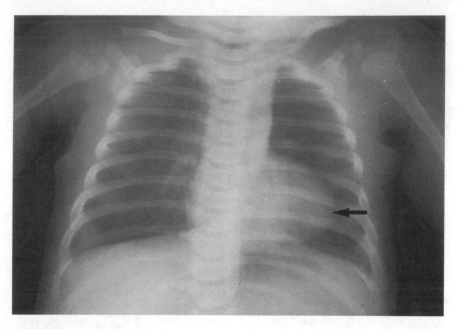

**Figure 12.**   *Fallot's tetralogy*

- Boot-shaped heart (arrow) due to right ventricular enlargement (apex is directed upwards and outwards).
- Paucity of lung vessels.
- This patient is a child but the same signs are found in adults. In this case the thymus overlies the enlarged aorta which cannot be seen.
- Check for a right aortic knuckle (present in 25% but not in this case).

1. Pulse and blood pressure. A low blood pressure and pulsus paradoxus are typical.
2. Jugular venous pressure. This is raised; Kussmaul's sign is rare. The $x$ and $y$ descents are prominent.
3. Apex beat. Impalpable.
4. Heart sounds. These are distant. There may be an early third heart sound and an early pericardial knock (as rapid ventricular filling is abruptly halted).
5. Hepatosplenomegaly, ascites and oedema provide an important clue.
6. Look for signs of the underlying aetiology (radiation, tumour, tuberculosis, connective tissue disease, chronic renal failure, trauma).

## Hypertrophic Cardiomyopathy

It is always important to consider this diagnosis—it is a popular 'trap'! The classical signs are:

1. Pulse. This is typically sharp rising and jerky, owing to rapid ejection by a hypertrophied ventricle early in systole, followed then by obstruction. It is not like the pulse of aortic stenosis.
2. Jugular venous pressure. There is a prominent $a$ wave, due to forceful atrial contraction against a non-compliant ventricle.
3. Apex beat. There is typically a double or triple impulse due to presystolic ventricular expansion following atrial contraction.
4. Auscultation:
   (a) late systolic ejection murmur (left sternal edge);
   (b) pansystolic murmur (apex) from mitral incompetence;
   (c) fourth heart sound.
   N.B. There are no diastolic murmurs.
5. Dynamic manoeuvres. The murmur is louder with the Valsalva manoeuvre, standing and isotonic exercise (e.g., jogging). The murmur is softer with squatting, raising the legs and isometric exercise (e.g., forceful hand grip).

Results of investigations:

1. Electrocardiogram:
   (a) left ventricular hypertrophy;
   (b) deep $Q$ waves;
   (c) conduction defects.
2. Chest X-ray film:
   (a) left ventricle enlarged with a hump along the border;
   (b) no valve calcification.
3. Echocardiogram:
   (a) ASH (asymmetrical hypertrophy of the ventricular septum);
   (b) SAM (systolic anterior motion of the mitral valve);
   (c) midsystolic closure of the aortic valve;
   (d) Doppler detection of mitral regurgitation.

## Non-cyanotic Congenital Heart Disease

These are difficult examination cases that can crop up in the test.

### Atrial Septal Defect (ASD)

There are two types.
1. Ostium secundum.
   This is the commonest and presents in adult life with:
   (a) fixed splitting of the second heart sound;
   (b) pulmonary systolic ejection murmur (increasing on inspiration);
   (c) pulmonary hypertension (late).

   Results of Investigations

   (a) Electrocardiogram
       (i)   right axis deviation;
       (ii)  right bundle branch block;
       (iii) right ventricular hypertrophy (systolic overload).
   (b) Chest X-ray film (p. 150)
       (i)   increased pulmonary vasculature;
       (ii)  enlarged right atrium and ventricle;
       (iii) dilated main pulmonary artery;
       (iv)  small aortic knob.
   (c) Echocardiogram
       (i)   paradoxical septal motion;
       (ii)  Echo drop-out in atrial septum;
       (iii) Doppler detection of shunt at atrial level.
   Indication for operation: Almost all need to be surgically closed when the left-to-right shunt is measured to be at least 1.5 to 1 (unless there is reversal of the shunt).
2. Ostium primum.
   This is an endocardial cushion defect adjacent to the atrioventricular valves. The signs are the same as for ostium secundum, but associated mitral incompetence, tricuspid incompetence or ventricular septal defect is common. The electrocardiogram is particularly helpful, as there is left axis deviation and right bundle branch block (and sometimes a prolonged P-R interval).
   Look also for the presence of Down's syndrome and skeletal upper limb defects (Holt-Oram syndrome).

### Ventricular Septal Defect (VSD)

The clues to the diagnosis of VSD are a thrill and a harsh pansystolic murmur at the left sternal edge. Sometimes mitral incompetence is also present. Down's syndrome is associated.

The electrocardiogram and chest X-ray film may show left ventricular hypertrophy. The chest X-ray film may also show increased pulmonary vasculature and an enlarged right ventricle. The echocardiogram will show the defect and detect the shunt.

Indication for operation: Closure is indicated when the left-to-right shunt is moderate to large, with the pulmonary-to-systemic flow being >1.5 to 1.

## Patent Ductus Arteriosus

In this condition there is a vessel from the bifurcation of the pulmonary artery to the aorta. The shunt is usually from aorta to pulmonary artery. Reversal of the shunt leads to differential cyanosis and clubbing (toes, NOT fingers). Often a continuous murmur is heard. Confusion with aortic stenosis and incompetence commonly occurs when candidates examine these patients.

Indication for operation: Diagnosis (unless there is pulmonary hypertension).

The electrocardiogram may show left ventricular hypertrophy (diastolic over-load).

Chest X-ray film may show increased pulmonary vasculature, calcification of the duct (trumpet-shaped calcification) and an enlarged left ventricle.

Echocardiography will demonstrate continuous flow in the main pulmonary artery.

## Coarctation of the Aorta

The commonest site for this lesion is just distal to the origin of the left subclavian artery.

Look for a better developed upper body, delayed pulses, hypertension in the arms only, chest collateral vessels, a midsystolic murmur over the praecordium and back and changes of hypertension in the fundi. Turner's syndrome may be associated in some cases.

1. The electrocardiogram may show left ventricular hypertrophy (systolic over-load).
2. The chest X-ray film may show (p. 151):
   (a) enlarged left ventricle;
   (b) enlarged left subclavian artery;
   (c) dilated ascending aorta;
   (d) aortic indentation;
   (e) aortic prestenotic and poststenotic dilatation;
   (f) rib notching—second to sixth ribs on the inferior border.
3. The Echocardiogram may show:
   (a) left ventricular hypertrophy;
   (b) coar ation shelf in descending aorta;
   (c) abnormal flow patterns in same area.

# Cyanotic Congenital Heart Disease

This is a very difficult area. You will probably not be expected to identify the lesion exactly.

The common causes of the problem in adults are:

1. Eisenmenger's syndrome. Pulmonary hypertension plus a large communication between the left and right circulations (e.g., ventricular septal defect, patent ductus arteriosus, atrial septal defect).

2. Tetralogy of Fallot.
3. Complex lesions, e.g., univentricular heart, Ebstein's anomaly (if there is an associated atrial septal defect with a right-to-left shunt).

You must decide while examining the patient whether pulmonary hypertension is present, as this distinguishes Eisenmenger's syndrome from tetralogy of Fallot.

### Eisenmenger's Syndrome

This syndrome may be found in older adults who had right-to-left shunting occur prior to the availability of open-heart surgery. The physical signs may include cyanosis, clubbing and polycythaemia. The jugular venous pressure pattern may have a dominant *a* wave and sometimes a prominent *v* wave. A right ventricular heave and a palpable pulmonary component of the second heart sound ($P_2$) may be found. On auscultation there may be a loud $P_2$, a fourth heart sound, pulmonary ejection click, pulmonary incompetence and sometimes tricuspid incompetence (but there may be no murmurs).

The signs all add up to pulmonary hypertension in a cyanosed patient.

To work out the level of the shunt, pay close attention to the second heart sound:

1. Wide fixed split—atrial septal defect.
2. Single second sound—ventricular septal defect.
3. Normal second sound or reversed splitting—patent ductus arteriosus (look for differential cyanosis).
4. The electrocardiogram may show:
   (a) right ventricular hypertrophy;
   (b) P pulmonale.
5. The chest X-ray film may show (p. 150):
   (a) right ventricle and right atrium enlarged;
   (b) pulmonary artery prominent;
   (c) increased hilar vascular markings but attenuated peripheral vessels;
   (d) heart is NOT boot shaped.

### Tetralogy of Fallot

There are 4 features:

1. Ventricular septal defect.
2. Right ventricular outflow obstruction (which determines severity).
3. Over-riding aorta.
4. Right ventricular hypertrophy.

The physical signs may include cyanosis, clubbing, polycythaemia, a right ventricular heave and a thrill at the left sternal edge, but not cardiomegaly. On auscultation there may be a single second heart sound ($A_2$) and a short pulmonary ejection murmur.

1. The electrocardiogram may show:
   (a) right ventricular hypertrophy;
   (b) right axis deviation.

**Table 8-6.**  *Causes of Hypertension*

**Essential** (>95%)

**Secondary** (<5%)
*Renal Disease:* Renovascular disease (renal artery atherosclerosis, fibromuscular disease,
aneurysm, vasculitis)
Diffuse renal disease

*Endocrine:*  Cushing's syndrome (especially glucocorticoid treatment)
17 and 11 beta hydroxylase defects
Conn's syndrome (primary aldosteronism)
Phaeochromocytoma
Acromegaly, myxoedema
The contraceptive pill

*Coarctation of the Aorta*

*Other:*  Polycythaemia rubra vera
Toxaemia of pregnancy
Neurogenic (increased intracranial pressure, lead poisoning, acute intermittent
porphyria)
Hypercalcaemia

N.B. Alcohol consumption and obesity are associated with essential hypertension.

2. The chest X-ray film may show (p. 152):
    (a) normal-sized heart with a boot shape (i.e., a left concavity where the pulmonary artery normally is situated plus a prominent elevated apex);
    (b) right ventricle enlarged;
    (c) decreased vascularity of lung vessels;
    (d) right-sided aortic knob, arch and descending aorta (25%).
3. The echocardiogram will demonstrate the anatomical abnormalities.

## Hypertensive Examination

This patient has hypertension. Please make an examination.

### Method

Stand back and inspect. Look for evidence of Cushing's syndrome (p. 190), acromegaly (p. 192), polycythaemia (p. 82) and uraemia (p. 113) (Table 8-6). If one of these is present, modify your examination in the appropriate way.

Next confirm that the blood pressure is elevated. Ask to measure it in both arms and also lying and standing. Measurement in the legs in a young patient is important.

Feel the radial pulse and very carefully feel for radiofemoral delay. Palpate for radial-radial asymmetry and inspect both hands for vasculitic changes.

Now look at the face. Inspect the conjunctivae for injection (polycythaemia), then examine the fundi for hypertensive changes (see Table 8-7). Describe what you see when presenting rather than just giving a grade.

**Table 8-7.** *Fundoscopy Changes in Hypertension*

| | |
|---|---|
| Grade I | Silver Wiring |
| Grade II | Above changes plus arteriovenous nipping |
| Grade III | Above changes plus haemorrhages (characteristically flame shaped) and exudates. Soft exudates, also called cottonwool spots, due to ischaemia; hard exudates due to lipid residues from leaky vessels. |
| Grade IV | Above changes plus papilloedema |

Examine the rest of the cardiovascular system, looking especially for left ventricular failure and coarctation of the aorta. Usually a fourth heart sound is present in severe hypertension.

The abdomen should be carefully examined (p. 165) for renal masses, adrenal masses and an abdominal aneurysm. Auscultate for renal bruits (due to fibromuscular dysplasia or atheroma). These usually have a diastolic component. Listen first just to the right or left of the midline above the umbilicus. Then sit the patient up and listen in the flanks (a systolic-diastolic bruit in the costovertebral area suggests a renal arteriovenous fistula). Ask at the end for the results of urine analysis (signs of renal disease). Also remember the possibility of cerebrovascular accidents, secondary to hypertension, causing other physical signs.

## Marfan's Syndrome

This patient has a heart murmur. Please make an examination.

### *Method*

Fortunately, you notice a Marfanoid habitus. While performing your normal cardiovascular examination look also for the following signs.

*Hands and arms.* Look for arachnodactyly (spider fingers) and joint hypermobility as well as long, thin limbs.

*Face.* You may notice a long and narrow face. Look for lens dislocation (the patient will be wearing thick spectacles). The sclerae may occasionally be blue. Look in the mouth for a high-arched palate.

*Chest.* Note any pectus carinatum or excavatum.

*Heart.* Auscultate for aortic incompetence and mitral valve prolapse. Also look for the signs of dissecting aneurysm or coarctation of the aorta.

*Back.* Look for kyphoscoliosis and hypermobility (p. 204).

Always ask at the end to measure the arm span, which will exceed the height. The upper segment to lower segment ratio will be less than 0.85 (the upper segment is from the crown to the symphysis pubis, whilst the lower segment is from the symphysis pubis to the ground).

**Table 8-8.** *Causes of Generalized Oedema*

1. Cardiac—congestive cardiac failure (p. 38), constrictive pericarditis (p. 147)
2. Hepatic—cirrhosis (p. 181)
3. Renal—nephrotic syndrome (Table 6-35, p. 114)
4. Malabsorption or starvation (p. 64)
5. Protein-losing enteropathy
6. Beri Beri ('wet')
7. Myxoedema (p. 188)
8. Cyclical oedema

# Oedema

This patient has oedema. Please make an assessment.

## *Method*

First stand back and look. Note whether the oedema is localized or generalized and whether it is gravitational or not.

Assess nutrition quickly (as hypoalbuminaemia and also beri beri due to vitamin $B_1$ deficiency can cause oedema). Also look for any obvious signs of myxoedema, which must never be missed.

Undress the patient and further define the areas affected. Palpate for pitting. Proceed, depending on your findings (Table 8-8).

## *1. Pitting Lower Limb Oedema*

Define the extent of the oedema and look for signs of deep venous thrombosis. Feel the inguinal nodes. Go to the abdomen and look for abdominal wall oedema, prominent abdominal wall veins (inferior vena caval obstruction), ascites, any abdominal masses and evidence of liver disease. A pulsatile liver (tricuspid incompetence) or malignant involvement should be particularly looked for. Examine next the jugular venous pressure. Then examine for signs of right ventricular failure and constrictive pericarditis. Feel all the node groups. Finally examine for delayed ankle jerks (to exclude hypothyroidism) and look at the urine analysis.

## *2. Non-Pitting Lower Limb Oedema*

Consider the various causes, including lymphoedema (from malignant infiltration, congenital disease, filariasis, Milroy's disease) and myxoedema.

## *3. Superior Vena Cava (SVC) Obstruction* (Table 8-9)

The patient may appear Cushingoid (p. 190), from either a tumour or treatment with steroids. Note the plethoric cyanosed face with periorbital oedema. There may be exophthalmos and conjunctival injection. A mass in the chest may have caused a Horner's syndrome (p. 209). Examine the fundi for venous dilatation. The neck is enlarged. The jugular venous pressure is raised, but the vein is not pul-

**Table 8-9.** *Causes of Superior Vena Caval Obstruction*

1. Lung Carcinoma (90%) (p. 51)
2. Retrosternal tumours, e.g., lymphoma (p. 87), thymoma (p. 124), dermoid
3. Retrosternal goitre (p. 185)
4. Massive mediastinal lymphadenopathy
5. Aortic aneurysm

satile. Decide if the thyroid gland is enlarged. Feel for supraclavicular lymphad-enopathy and listen over the trachea for inspiratory stridor. Examine the chest carefully for distended venous collaterals. One or both arms may be oedematous. Look for all the peripheral manifestations of lung carcinoma.

# THE RESPIRATORY SYSTEM

## Respiratory Examination

This patient presented with breathlessness. Please examine her.

### *Method* (Figure 13)

Undress the patient to the waist and sit her over the side of the bed. Whilst standing back to make your usual inspection, ask if sputum is available for you to look at. A large volume of purulent sputum is an important clue to bronchiec-tasis (p. 48). Haemoptysis suggests lung carcinoma or pulmonary infection. Look for evidence of dyspnoea at rest and count the respiratory rate. Note the use of the accessory muscles of respiration and any intercostal indrawing of the lower ribs anteriorly (an important sign of emphysema). General cachexia should also be noted.

Pick up the hands. Note clubbing (Table 8-10), peripheral cyanosis, nicotine staining and anaemia, and look for wasting of the small muscles of the hands and weakness of finger abduction (which may be due to a lower trunk brachial plexus lesion from apical lung carcinoma involvement). Palpate the wrists for tenderness if there is clubbing (hypertrophic pulmonary osteoarthropathy [HPO]). While holding the hand palpate the radial pulse for obvious pulsus paradoxus.

Go on to the face. Look closely at the eyes for ptosis and constriction of the pupils and if indicated palpate the forehead for loss of sweating (Horner's syn-drome [p. 209]). Inspect the tongue for central cyanosis.

Palpate the position of the trachea. This is a most important sign, so spend time on it. If the trachea is displaced, you must concentrate on the upper lobes for physical signs. Also note the presence of a tracheal tug, which indicates gross overexpansion of the chest with airflow obstruction. Now ask the patient to cough and note whether this is a loose cough, a dry cough or a bovine cough indicating possible recurrent laryngeal nerve palsy. Next measure the forced expiratory time (FET). Tell the patient to take a maximal inspiration and blow out as rapidly and

**Figure 13.**  *Respiratory System*

Sitting up

GENERAL INSPECTION
    Sputum mug contents (blood, pus, etc.)
    Type of cough
    Rate and depth of respiration
    Accessory muscles of respiration

FACE
    Eyes—Horner's syndrome (apical
        tumour), jaundice, anaemia
    Mouth—central cyanosis
    Voice—hoarseness (recurrent
        laryngeal nerve palsy)

HANDS
    Clubbing
    Cyanosis (peripheral)
    Nicotine staining
    Wasting, weakness—finger abduction
    Wrist tenderness (HPO)
    Pulse (tachycardia; pulsus paradoxus)
    Flapping tremor ($CO_2$ narcosis)

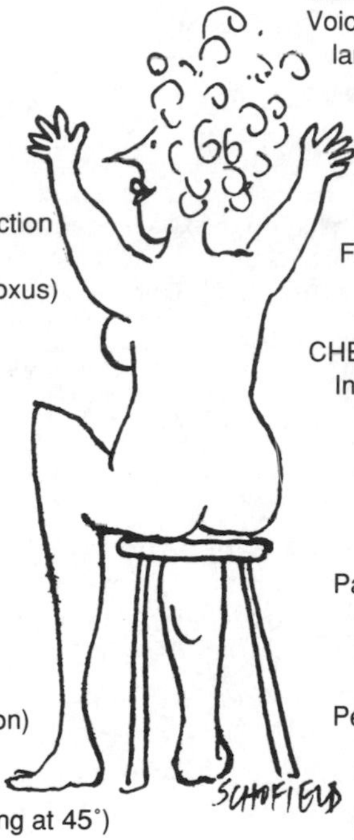

TRACHEA

FORCED EXPIRATORY TIME

CHEST ANTERIORLY
    Inspect
    Palpate
        Supraclavicular nodes
        Vocal fremitis
        Axillary nodes
        Breasts
    Percuss
    Auscultate
    Pemberton's sign (SVC obstruction)

CHEST POSTERIORLY
    Inspect
        Shape of chest and spine
        Scars
        Radiotherapy marks
        Prominent veins (determine
            direction of flow)
    Palpate
        Cervical lymph nodes
        Expansion
        Vocal fremitus
    Percuss
        Supraclavicular region
        Back
        Axillae
        Tidal percussion (diaphragm)
    Auscultate
        Breath sounds
        Adventitial sounds
        Vocal resonance

CARDIOVASCULAR SYSTEM (Lying at 45°)
    Jugular venous pressure
        (SVC obstruction, etc.)
    Apex beat
    Pulmonary hypertension
    Cor pulmonale

SCHOFIELD

OTHER
    Temperature chart (infection)
    Fundi ($CO_2$ narcosis)
    Evidence of malignancy or pleural
        effusion: examine breasts, abdomen,
        rectal exam, lymph nodes, etc.

HPO = hypertrophic pulmonary osteoarthropathy.
SVC = superior vena cava.

**Table 8-10.**   *Causes of Clubbing*

1. Respiratory
   a) lung carcinoma (usually *not* small cell carcinoma) (p. 51) or carcinoid tumour
   b) chronic pulmonary suppuration (e.g., bronchiectasis, lung abscess, empyema)
      (p. 48)
   c) idiopathic pulmonary fibrosis, asbestosis (p. 56)
   d) cystic fibrosis (p. 61)
   e) pleural fibroma or benign fibrous mesothelioma
   f) mediastinal disease, e.g., thymoma, lymphoma, carcinoma
2. Cardiovascular
   a) infective endocarditis (p. 33)
   b) cyanotic congenital heart disease (p. 155)
3. Other
   a) inflammatory bowel disease (p. 68)
   b) cirrhosis (p. 72)
   c) coeliac disease (p. 68)
   d) thyrotoxicosis (p. 187)
   e) brachial arteriovenous aneurysm or axillary artery aneurysm (unilateral)
   f) neurogenic diaphragmatic tumours
   g) familial (usually before puberty) or idiopathic
   h) pregnancy

N.B.  Clubbing does *not* occur with chronic obstructive pulmonary disease, sarcoidosis, extrinsic allergic
      alveolitis or coal workers' pneumoconiosis or silicosis. With this important sign decide if it is definitely
      present or absent. Don't call it 'early' if in doubt about it.

completely as possible. Note audible wheeze. Prolongation of expiration beyond
three seconds is evidence of chronic airflow limitation.

The next step is to examine the chest. You may wish to examine this anteriorly
first, or go around to the back initially. The advantage of the latter is that there are
usually more signs there, unless the trachea is obviously displaced.

Inspect the back. Look for kyphoscoliosis. Don't miss ankylosing spondylitis
(p. 204), which causes decreased chest expansion and upper lobe fibrosis. Look
for thoracotomy scars and prominent veins. Also note any skin changes from
radiotherapy.

Palpate first the cervical nodes from behind. Then examine for expansion—first
upper lobe expansion, which is best seen by looking over the patient's shoulders
at clavicular movement during moderate respiration. The affected side will show
a delay or decreased movement. Then examine lower lobe expansion by palpation.
Note asymmetry and reduction of movement.

Now ask the patient to bring her elbows together in front of her to move the
scapulae out of the way. Examine for vocal fremitus. Then percuss the back of the
chest and include both axillae. Do not miss a pleural effusion (Table 8-11).

Auscultate the chest. Note breath sounds (whether bronchial or vesicular) and
their intensity (normal or reduced) (Table 8-12). Listen for adventitial sounds
(crackles and wheezes) (Table 8-13). Finally examine for vocal resonance. If a
localized abnormality is found, try to determine the abnormal segment.

Return to the front of the chest. Inspect again for chest deformity, symmetry of

**Table 8-11.**   *Pleural Effusion*

*Causes:*
1. Transudate (protein <30g/L, pleural/serum protein <0.5, lactate dehydrogenase (LDH <200U/L, pleural/serum LDH <0.6)
   (a) cardiac failure
   (b) nephrotic syndrome
   (c) liver failure
   (d) Meigs' syndrome (ovarian fibroma and effusion)
   (e) hypothyroidism
2. Exudate (protein >30g/L, pleural/serum protein >0.5, lactate dehydrogenase (LDH) >200U/L, pleural/serum LDH >0.6)
   (a) pneumonia
   (b) neoplasm—lung carcinoma, metastatic carcinoma, mesothelioma
   (c) tuberculosis
   (d) pulmonary infarction
   (e) subphrenic abscess
   (f) pancreatitis
   (g) connective tissue disease, e.g., rheumatoid arthritis, systemic lupus erythematosus
   (h) drugs, e.g., nitrofurantoin (acute), methysergide (chronic); drugs causing lupus (p. 100), chemotherapeutic agents, bromocryptine
   (i) radiation

*Pleural fluid analysis: differential diagnosis*

| | |
|---|---|
| pH <7.2 | Empyema, tuberculosis, neoplasm, rheumatoid arthritis, oesophageal rupture |
| Glucose <3.33mmol/L | Infection, carcinoma, mesothelioma, rheumatoid arthritis |
| Red blood cells >5000/µL | Pulmonary infarction, neoplasm, trauma, asbestosis, tuberculosis, pancreatitis |
| Amylase >2000U/L | Pancreatitis, abdominal viscera rupture, oesophageal rupture |
| Complement decreased | Rheumatoid arthritis, systemic lupus erythematosus |
| Chylous | Tumour (usually lymphoma), thoracic duct trauma, tuberculosis, tuberous sclerosis |

chest wall movement, distended veins, radiotherapy changes and scars. Palpate the supraclavicular nodes carefully. Palpate the apex beat and measure chest expansion. Then test for vocal fremitus and proceed with percussion and auscultation as before. Listen high up in the axillae too. Before leaving the chest, feel the axillary nodes and breasts.

Lie the patient down at 45 degrees and visually measure the jugular venous pressure. Then examine the praecordium for signs of pulmonary hypertension and cor pulmonale. Finally examine the liver and look for peripheral oedema. Check for Pemberton's sign if indicated (p. 185).

Before leaving the patient, ask if you may see the temperature chart.

## Chest X-ray Films

*Hints on how to read a chest X-ray*

This is a very valuable investigation and some even consider a chest X-ray an extension of the physical examination. It is essential to be familiar with the

**Table 8-12.** *Breath Sounds*

1. *Vesicular.* Normal, likened to wind rustling in the leaves.
2. *Bronchial.* The expiratory phase is prolonged and has a blowing quality. The breath sounds heard over the trachea and right and left main bronchi are sometimes rather bronchial in quality.
   Causes:
   a) lobar pneumonia (common)
   b) localized fibrosis or collapse
   c) above a pleural effusion
   d) large lung cavity
3. *Reduced.* Use this term rather than 'air entry'.
   Causes:
   a) emphysema
   b) large lung mass
   c) collapse, fibrosis or pneumonia
   d) effusion
   e) pneumothorax

**Table 8-13.** *Added Sounds*

1. **Wheezes (Rhonchi)**
   Inspiratory wheezes—characteristic of asthma or upper airway extrathoracic obstruction
   Expiratory wheezes—occur in asthma and chronic obstructive pulmonary disease
   Fixed inspiratory wheeze (monophonic—does not change with respiration). An important sign of fixed bronchial obstruction, usually due to a carcinoma
2. **Crackles (Crepitations)**
   Late or pan–inspiratory crackles:
   Fine—caused by fibrosis—dry crackles (p. 56)
   Medium—caused by left ventricular failure (p. 38)
   Coarse—caused by bronchiectasis or retained secretions (p. 48)
   Early inspiratory crackles: (coarse)—caused by chronic obstructive pulmonary disease
       (p. 54)

various radiographic appearances. As a physician, one should feel personally responsible for viewing all the patient's radiographs.

When first viewing the chest radiograph check:

1. Film date.
2. Type of film—postero-anterior (PA) or antero–posterior (AP) film; the latter (which may be labelled 'portable') magnifies heart size making assessment of cardiac diameter difficult.
3. Correct orientation—the left side is most reliably determined by the position of stomach gas.
4. Film 'centring'—the medial ends of each clavicle should be equidistant from the spines of the vertebrae. Rotation affects mediastinal and hilar shadows, causing undue prominence on the side opposite to which the patient was turned.

Next, systematically examine the PA film, comparing right and left sides carefully for abnormalities of:

1. Soft tissues (e.g., mastectomy, subcutaneous emphysema) and bony skeleton (e.g., rib fractures, malignant deposits)
2. Tracheal displacement, paratracheal masses.
3. Heart size, borders and retrocardiac density.
4. Aorta and upper mediastinum (count ribs, look for mediastinal shift)
5. Diaphragm (right higher than left by 1 to 3cm normally), cardiophrenic and costophrenic angles.
6. Lung hila (left normally above right by up to 3cm, usually no larger than an average thumb).
7. Lung fields—upper zone (to lower border of second rib), mid-zone (from upper zone to lower border fourth rib) and lower zone (from mid-zone to diaphragm).
8. Pleura.
9. Gastric bubble (normally there should be no opacity >0.5cm above the air bubble).

Learn to do all this rapidly and accurately.

Finally, always ask to look at a lateral film. Examine it just as carefully. The lateral film is used to help decide the exact anatomical site of an abnormality. Candidates must learn the normal position of the fissures (the horizontal fissure, seen sometimes on the PA and lateral, is a fine horizontal line at the level of the fourth costal cartilage; while the oblique fissure is only seen sometimes on the lateral, beginning at the level of the fifth thoracic vertebra and running downwards to the diaphragm at the junction of its anterior and middle thirds). The lung segments must also be memorized (Figure 14). Remember, abnormalities in the lung fields are described by terms such as 'mottling', 'opacity' or 'shadow'—it is usually unwise to attempt to make a precise diagnosis of the underlying pathology in your initial assessment of the chest X-ray (Table 8-14).

*Some Common Radiological Abnormalities*

In this section, a few selected films of important conditions are presented. As well, the differential diagnosis of some common diagnostic lung radiological abnormalities are tabled. Practise looking at films—it will pay great dividends!

# THE GASTROINTESTINAL SYSTEM

Please examine this patient's abdomen.

## *Method* (Figure 23)

Position the patient correctly, with one pillow for the head and complete exposure of the abdomen.

Briefly look at the patient's general appearance and inspect particularly for signs of chronic liver disease and renal disease.

Inspect the abdomen now from the side, squatting to the patient's level. Large masses may be visible. Ask the patient to take slow, deep breaths. Now stand up

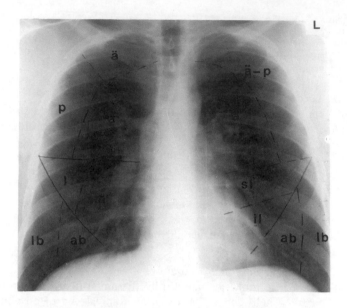

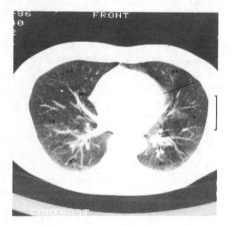

**Figure 14.** *The lung segments*

(Top left) Postero-anterior view, (bottom left) CT scan through lung bases, (top right) Left lateral view, (bottom right) right lateral view.

**Right upper lobe:** ä = apical segment; a = anterior segment, p = posterior segment. **Left upper lobe:** ä — p = apico-posterior segment, a = anterior segment, sl = superior lingular segment, il = inferior lingular segment. **Right middle lobe (rml):** m = medial segment, l = lateral segment. **Right lower lobe:** äl = apical segment, mb = medial basal segment, lb = lateral basal segment, ab = anterior basal segment, pb = posterior basal segment. **Left lower lobe**: äl = apical segment, lb = lateral basal segment, ab = anterior basal segment, pb = posterior basal segment.

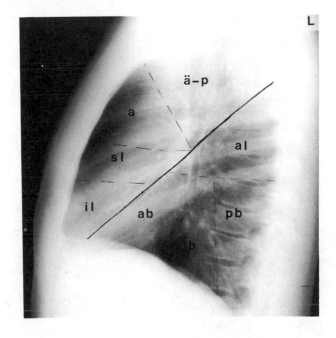

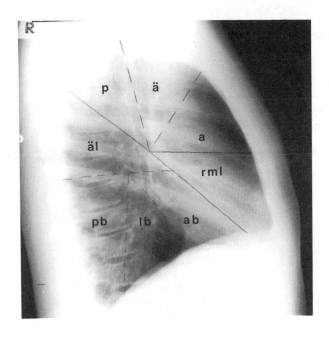

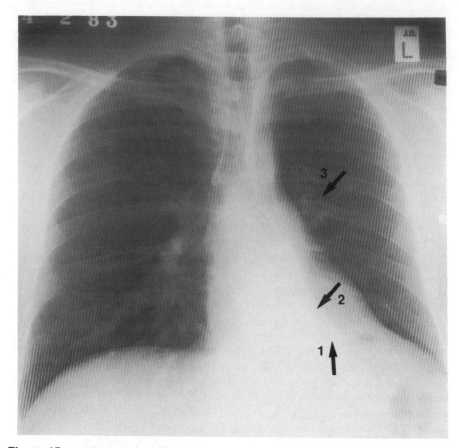

**Figure 15.**  *Left lower lobe collapse*

- Loss of left hemidiaphragm outline contour or contrast (arrow 1).
- Dense triangular shadow projected behind the heart ('sail sign') (arrow 2).
- Left hilum depressed (arrow 3).
- Paucity of left lung vessels compared to the right.
- This is a commonly missed diagnosis—for the left lower lobe collapse to be seen, the thoracic spine must be visualized as it should be in a correctly exposed film; the collapse will be better seen in an over-penetrated film.

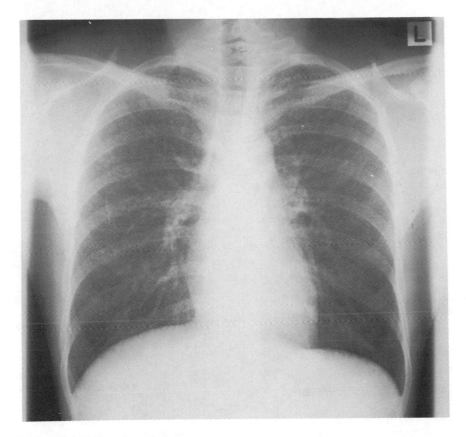

**Figure 16.**   *Miliary tuberculosis*

- There are multiple fine discrete nodules of soft tissue density uniformly distributed throughout both lung fields due to haematological dissemination.
- This condition does not cause miliary calcification.

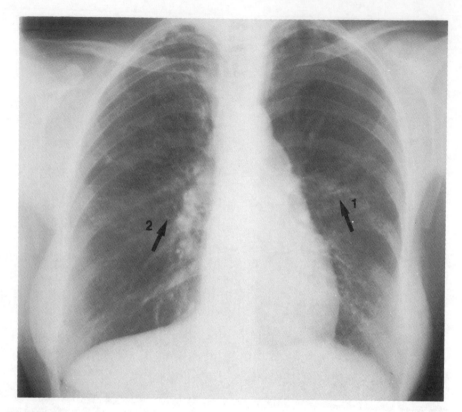

**Figure 17.** *Bronchiectasis*

- Tram-line shadows outline a bronchial course (arrow 1).
- Thickened circular shadows indicate dilated end-on bronchi (arrow 2).
- This is an example of proximal bronchiectasis due to bronchopulmonary aspergillosis.

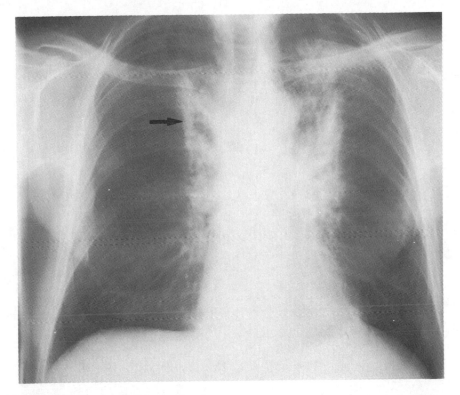

**Figure 18.**  *Upper and mid-zone fibrosis*

- Dense interstitial shadowing is seen in the medial parts of the upper and mid-zones bilaterally.
- This is an example of radiation-induced pulmonary fibrosis—the straight edge (arrow) corresponds to the limit of the radiation field.
- Underlying hilar and mediastinal lymphadenopathy is difficult to assess in the presence of this dense adjacent fibrosis—serial films and CT scans can be helpful.

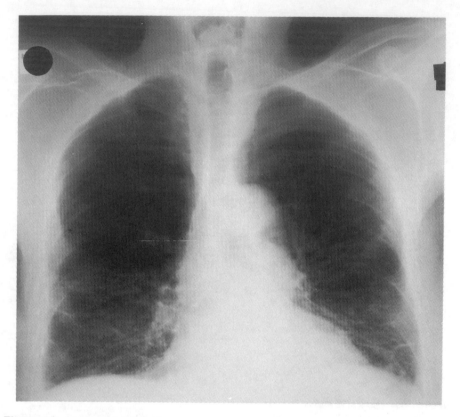

**Figure 19.**  *Lower zone fibrosis*

• Increased interstitial linear shadows are seen bilaterally.

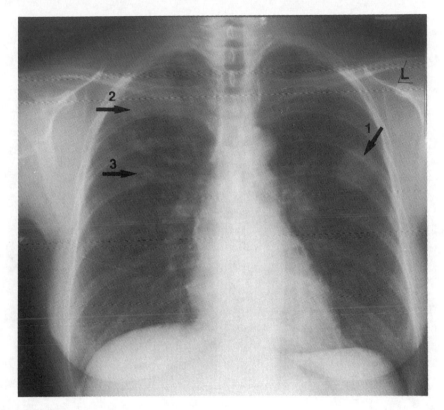

**Figure 20.**   *Coin lesion*

- There is a 3cm left mid-zone 'coin lesion' (arrow 1).
- The patient has right upper zone fibrosis (arrow 2) and granulomata (arrow 3) due to coincidental tuberculosis (these appearances were unchanged on serial films).

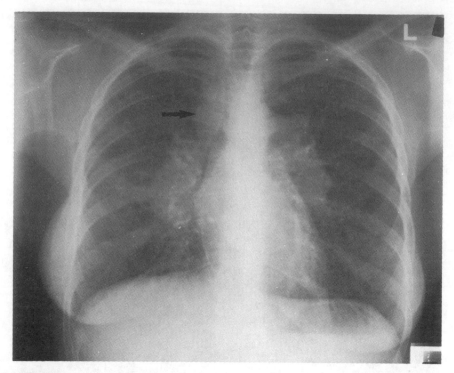

**Figure 21.**   *Bilateral hilar lymphadenopathy*

- Hila are enlarged (this is not due to vascular structures—see Figure 10).
- There is right para-tracheal enlargement (arrow).
- Minimal parenchymal infiltrate is present in the mid and lower zones.
- This is an example of sarcoidosis with bilateral hilar and right para-tracheal lymphadenopathy.

*Differential diagnosis of bilateral hilar lymphadenopathy*
1. Sarcoidosis.
2. Lymphoma, lymphatic leukaemia.
3. Metastases.
4. Infectious mononucleosis.

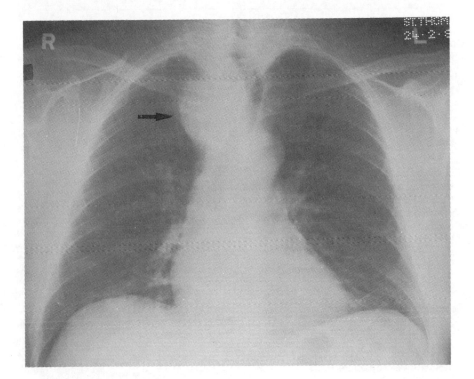

**Figure 22.** *Retrosternal mass*

- Widening of the superior mediastinum (arrow).
- Mass is causing tracheal displacement.

*Differential diagnosis (the 5 't's)*
1. Thyroid (retrosternal goitre).
2. Thymoma.
3. Teratoma.
4. 'Terrible' lymphoma or carcinoma.
5. Tortuous vessels, aortic aneurysm.

**Table 8-14.** *Differential Diagnosis of Radiological Appearances in Chest X-ray Film*

**Homogeneous Opacity**
Pneumonia—lobar or segmental
Collapse (p. 168)
Effusion

**Localized Non-homogeneous Opacity**
Pneumonia
Pulmonary infarct
Carcinoma
Tuberculosis

**Diffuse Opacities**
Miliary (<2mm): (p. 169)
   Miliary tuberculosis
   Miliary metastases (especially breast, thyroid, melanoma, pancreas)
   Sarcoidosis
   Pneumoconiosis
   Lymphoma
   Lymphangitis
   Viral pneumonia
   Vasculitis, e.g., polyarteritis

Nodular (3 to 10mm)
   Pneumonia
   Pneumoconiosis
   Tuberculosis
   Metastatic carcinoma
   Sarcoidosis

**Reticular (linear opacities)**
Fibrosis (p. 171)

**Cavitated Lesion**
Lung abscess
Carcinoma (usually squamous cell) or Hodgkin's disease
Tuberculosis
Fungi, e.g., coccidiodomycosis

**Calcified Lesions in the Lung Fields**
Tuberculosis
Pneumoconiosis
Post chicken pox pneumonia
Tularaemia

**Miliary Calcification**
Post chicken pox pneumonia
Histoplasmosis
Coccidiodomycosis
Ectopic calcification in renal failure, hyperparathyroidism

**Coin Lesion (p. 173)**
Carcinoma (primary or metastatic—look closely for any rib lesion)
Tuberculoma
Hamartoma
Granuloma (e.g. fungus)
Arteriovenous fistula
Rheumatoid nodule
Lung abscess
Hydatid cyst

**Figure 23.** *Gastrointestinal System*

Lying flat (1 pillow)

GENERAL INSPECTION
Jaundice (liver disease, etc.)
Pigmentation (e.g., haemochromatosis)
Xanthomata (e.g., primary biliary cirrhosis, chronic biliary tract obstruction)
Mental state (encephalopathy)

FACE
Eyes—Sclera: jaundice, anaemia, iritis
  —Cornea: Kayser-Fleischer rings (Wilson's disease)
Parotids (alcohol)
Mouth—Breath: fetor hepaticus
  —Lips: stomatitis, leukoplakia, ulceration, localized pigmentation (Peutz-Jegher syndrome), telangiectasia (hereditary haemorrhagic telangiectasia)
  —Gums: gingivitis, bleeding, hypertrophy, pigmentation, monilia
  —Tongue: atrophic glossitis, leukoplakia, ulceration

CERVICAL/AXILLARY LYMPH NODES

CHEST
Gynaecomastia
Spider naevi

HANDS
Nails—Clubbing
  —Leukonychia (white nails)
Palmar Erythema
Dupuytren's contractures (alcohol)
Arthropathy
Hepatic flap

GROIN
Genitalia
Lymph nodes
Hernial orifices (standing up and coughing)

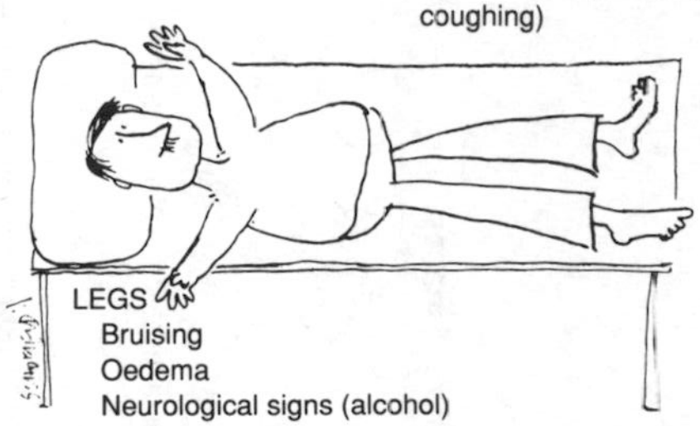

LEGS
Bruising
Oedema
Neurological signs (alcohol)

OTHER
Rectal examination—inspect (fistulae, tags, blood on glove, etc.), palpate (masses)
Urine analysis (bile, etc.)
Blood pressure (renal disease)
Cardiovascular system (cardiomyopathy)
Neurological system (Wernicke's encephalopathy, etc.)
Temperature chart (infection)

ARMS
Spider naevi
Bruising
Wasting
Scratch marks (chronic cholestasis)

ABDOMEN
Inspect
  Scars
  Distension
  Prominent veins—determine direction of flow (Caput Medusae; inferior vena caval obstruction)
  Striae
  Bruising
  Localized masses
  Visible peristalsis
Palpate
  Superficial palpation—tenderness, rigidity, outline of any mass
  Deep palpation—organomegaly (liver, gallbladder, spleen, kidney), abnormal masses
  Roll onto right side (spleen)
Percuss
  Viscera outline
  Ascites—shifting dullness
Auscultate
  Bowel sounds
  Bruits, hums
  Rubs

**Table 8-15.**   *Differential Diagnosis in Liver Palpation*

**Hepatomegaly**
1. Massive
   a) Metastases
   b) Alcoholic liver disease with fatty infiltration
   c) Myeloproliferative disease (p. 84)
   d) Right heart failure (p. 38)
   e) Hepatoma
2. Moderate
   a) The above causes
   b) Haemochromatosis
   c) Haematological disease, e.g., chronic myeloid leukaemia, lymphoma (p. 87)
   d) Fatty liver, e.g., diabetes mellitus, toxins
3. Mild
   a) The above causes
   b) Hepatitis (viral, drugs)
   c) Cirrhosis
   d) Biliary obstruction
   e) Granulomatous disorders
   f) Hydatid disease
   g) Amyloid and other infiltrative diseases
   h) HIV infection
   i) Ischaemia

**Firm and Irregular Liver**
1. Cirrhosis
2. Metastatic disease
3. Hydatid disease, granuloma, amyloid, cysts, lipidoses

**Tender Liver**
1. Hepatitis
2. Rapid liver enlargement, e.g., right heart failure, Budd-Chiari syndrome (p. 76)
3. Hepatoma

**Pulsatile Liver**
1. Tricuspid incompetence (p. 147)
2. Hepatoma
3. Vascular abnormalities

and look for scars, distension, prominent veins, striae, bruising and pigmentation.

Palpate lightly in each quadrant for masses (Tables 8-15 to 8-20). Ask first if any particular area is tender (to avoid causing pain and also to obtain a clue to the site of possible pathology). Next palpate more deeply in each quadrant and then specifically feel for hepatomegaly and splenomegaly. A palpable liver may be due to enlargement or ptosis. If there is hepatomegaly (Table 8-15), confirm with percussion and estimate the span (normal span approximately 12.5cm). The same procedure is followed for splenomegaly (Table 8-19). Always roll the patient on to the right side and palpate again if no spleen is palpable.

Carefully feel for the kidneys bimanually. Remember that any left-sided mass

**Table 8-16.** *Causes of Renal Masses*

**Bilateral:**
1. Polycystic kidneys (Table 8-17)
2. Hydronephrosis or pyonephrosis (bilateral)
3. Hypernephroma (bilateral renal cell carcinoma)
4. Diabetic nephropathy (early)
5. Nephrotic syndrome (Table 6-35)
6. Acute renal vein thrombosis (bilateral)
7. Amyloid, lymphoma and other infiltrative diseases
8. Acromegaly

**Unilateral:**
1. Renal cell carcinoma
2. Hydronephrosis or pyonephrosis
3. Polycystic kidney (asymmetrical enlargement)
4. Acute renal vein thrombosis
5. Normal right kidney or a solitary kidney (uncommon)

**Table 8-17.** *Adult Polycystic Kidneys*

If you find polycystic kidneys remember these very important points:
1. Take the blood pressure (75% have hypertension).
2. Examine the urine for haematuria (due to haemorrhage into a cyst) and proteinuria (usually less than 2g/day when measured).
3. Look for evidence of anaemia (due to chronic renal failure) or polycythaemia (due to high erythropoietin levels). Note the haemoglobin level is higer than expected for the degree of renal failure.
4. Note the presence of hepatic (30%) and splenic cysts (rare). These may cause confusion when examining the abdomen.

N.B. Subarachnoid haemorrhage occurs in 3% of patients due to intracranial aneurysm. As this is an autosomal dominant condition, all family members of patients with polycystic kidney disease without a history of subarachnoid haemorrhage should also be assessed.

may arise from a number of sites. Always consider, if you have found hepatosplenomegaly, the possibility of associated polycystic kidneys (a common trap for young players in the test).

The usual distinguishing features of a spleen as opposed to a kidney are:

1. The spleen has no palpable upper border.
2. The spleen has a notch.
3. The spleen moves inferomedially on respiration.
4. There is usually no resonance over a splenic mass.
5. The spleen is not bimanually palpable (i.e., not 'ballottable').
6. A friction rub may occasionally be heard over the spleen.

Percuss for ascites as a routine. If the abdomen is resonant on percussion out to the flanks, do not roll the patient over. Otherwise, look for shifting dullness. The technique is usually performed by percussing away from your side of the bed

**Table 8-18.** *Some Other Causes of Abdominal Masses*

**Right Iliac Fossa**
Appendicael abscess
Carcinoma of the caecum
Crohn's disease
Pelvic kidney
Ovarian tumour or cyst
Carcinoid tumour
Amoebiasis
Psoas abscess
Ileo-caecal tuberculosis

**Left Iliac Fossa**
Faeces (N.B. Can be indented)
Carcinoma of sigmoid or descending colon
Diverticular disease
Ovarian tumour or cyst
Psoas abscess

**Upper Abdomen**
Retroperitoneal lymphadenopathy (e.g., lymphoma, teratoma)
Abdominal aortic aneurysm (pulsatile)
Carcinoma of stomach
Pancreatic pseudocyst or tumour
Pyloric stenosis
Carcinoma of transverse colon

**Table 8-19.** *Causes of Splenomegaly*

1. Massive
   a) chronic myeloid leukaemia
   b) myelofibrosis
   c) primary lymphoma of spleen, hairy cell disease, malaria, kalar-azar (all rare)
2. Moderate
   a) the above causes
   b) portal hypertension (p. 76)
   c) lymphoma (p. 87)
   d) leukaemia (chronic or acute)
   e) thalassaemia (p. 80)
   f) storage diseases, e.g., Gaucher's disease
3. Small
   a) the above causes
   b) other myeloproliferative disorders—polycythaemia rubra vera (p. 82), essential
      thrombocythaemia
   c) haemolytic anaemia (p. 80)
   d) megaloblastic anaemia (rarely)
   e) infection, e.g., viral (infectious mononucleosis, hepatitis), bacterial (infective endocarditis)
   f) connective tissue disease or vasculitis, e.g., rheumatoid arthritis (p. 92), systemic lupus
      erythematosus (p. 97), polyarteritis nodosa
   g) infiltration, e.g., amyloidosis, sarcoidosis (p. 58)

N.B. Secondary carcinomatosis is a rare cause of splenomegaly.

**Table 8-20.**  *Causes of Hepatosplenomegaly*

1. Chronic liver disease with portal hypertension
2. Haematological disease, e.g., myeloproliferative disease, lymphoma, leukaemia, pernicious anaemia, sickle cell anaemia
3. Infection, e.g., acute viral hepatitis, infectious mononucleosis, cytomegalovirus
4. Infiltration, e.g., amyloid, sarcoid
5. Connective tissue disease, e.g., systemic lupus erythematosus
6. Acromegaly (p. 192)
7. Thyrotoxicosis (p. 187)

until you reach a dull note, then rolling the patient towards yourself and waiting at least a short time before percussing again for resonance.

Always auscultate briefly over the liver, spleen and renal areas. Listen for bruits, rubs and a venous hum. Note the presence of bowel sounds. An arterial systolic bruit over the liver is usually caused by either hepatocellular carcinoma or acute alcoholic hepatitis. A friction rub over the liver may be due to tumour, recent liver biopsy, infarction or gonococcal perihepatitis; splenic rubs indicate infarction. A venous hum occurs uncommonly in portal hypertension.

Examine the groins next. Palpate for inguinal lymphadenopathy. The testes must always be palpated.

If you now suspect liver disease, you must go on and look for the peripheral stigmata of chronic liver disease. In this instance, it is probably better to proceed from the abdomen to the chest wall. Look for gynaecomastia, spider naevi, hair loss (in males) and breast atrophy (in females). Examine the breasts if you suspect intra-abdominal malignant disease.

Sit the patient at 45 degrees and visually measure the jugular venous pressure so as not to miss constrictive pericarditis as a cause of cirrhosis. Palpate anteriorly for supraclavicular nodes, then sit the patient forwards and feel posteriorly for the other cervical nodes. Look at the back for sacral oedema and spider naevi. If ascites is present, ask permission to examine the chest for pleural effusions.

Look at the face next. Note any scleral abnormality (jaundice, anaemia or iritis) and look at the corneas for Kayser-Fleischer rings (Wilson's disease seems common in Adelaide, so be very careful to look for the presence of these rings if in that capital city). Xanthelasma are common in patients with primary biliary cirrhosis. Feel for parotid enlargement, which may be present soon after an acute alcoholic binge. Inspect the mouth with a torch and spatula for angular stomatitis, ulceration and atrophic glossitis. Smell the breath for fetor hepaticus.

Look at the arms for bruising and spider naevi. Next examine the hands. Ask the patient to extend his arms and hands and look for evidence of hepatic flap. Look also at the nails for clubbing and white nails, and note any palmar erythema and Dupuytren's contractures (the latter are associated with alcohol or trauma). The arthropathy of haemochromatosis may also be present (a degenerative arthritis that particularly involves the second and third metacarpophalangeal joints).

Next examine the legs for oedema and bruising. Look for the nervous system signs of alcoholism—namely, peripheral neuropathy, proximal myopathy, cerebellar syndrome, Wernicke's encephalopathy (bilateral VI nerve palsy, p. 216) and Korsakoff's psychosis.

Candidates are almost always stopped well before this stage. Don't forget to ask to perform a rectal examination and urine analysis. Also ask to look at the temperature chart. Examine for hernias by asking the patient to stand and cough.

If on the other hand you have found signs consistent with a haematological problem, proceed as described in that section.

If you find a pulsatile liver, examine the cardiovascular system (p. 135) and particularly note any signs of tricuspid incompetence.

If an enlarged kidney is present (Table 8-16), ask to check the blood pressure and the urine. If malignant disease is suspected, examine all the node groups, the lungs and the breasts after a thorough abdominal examination. Non-haematological malignant disease which causes hepatomegaly rarely leads to splenomegaly unless the portal vein is directly involved.

Haemochromatosis, an autosomal recessive disorder, is an important cause of liver disease and is common in the examination (p. 77). Consider this diagnosis if any of the following signs are present:

1. Pigmentation (bronze).
2. Arthropathy (typically degenerative arthritis of the metacarpophalangeal joints of the index and middle finger, but may involve any other joint; pseudogout may occur).
3. Testicular atrophy (due to iron deposition in the pituitary gland).
4. Dilated cardiomyopathy.
5. Glycosuria (due to diabetes mellitus).

N.B. If you are asked to examine the 'gastrointestinal system' rather than the 'abdomen', begin by examining the hands and go on to the arms, face, chest, abdomen and legs as described (Figure 23).

# THE HAEMATOLOGICAL SYSTEM

Please examine this patient's haemopoietic system.

## Haemopoietic Examination

### Method (Figure 24)

Position the patient as for a gastrointestinal examination (p. 165). Make sure he or she is fully undressed. Look for bruising, pigmentation, cyanosis, jaundice, scratch marks (due to myeloproliferative disease or lymphoma) and leg ulceration. Also note the presence of frontal bossing and the racial origin of the patient (thalassaemia is more common in Asian or Greek races).

Pick up the patient's hands. Look at the nails for koilonychia (spoon-shaped nails which are rarely seen today and indicate iron deficiency) and the changes of

**Figure 24.** *Haematological System*

Lying flat (1 pillow)

GENERAL INSPECTION
Bruising (thrombocytopenia, scurvy, etc.)
—Petechiae (pin head bleeding)
—Ecchymoses (large bruises)
Pigmentation (lymphoma)
Rashes and infiltrative lesions (lymphoma)
Ulceration (neutropenia)
Cyanosis (polycythaemia)
Plethora (polycythaemia)
Jaundice (haemolysis)
Scratch marks (myeloproliferative
   disease)
Racial origin

CERVICAL NODES (Sitting up)
Palpate from behind

BONY TENDERNESS
Sternum
Clavicles
Shoulders
Spine

HANDS
Nails—koilonychia
Palm crease pallor (anaemia)
Arthropathy (haemophilia;
   secondary gout; drug treatment, etc.)
Pulse

ABDOMEN (Lying flat) and GENITALIA
Detailed examination (p. 177)

INGUINAL NODES

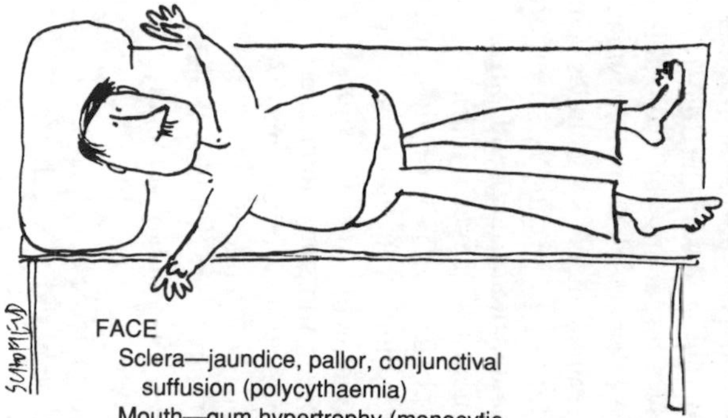

FACE
Sclera—jaundice, pallor, conjunctival
   suffusion (polycythaemia)
Mouth—gum hypertrophy (monocytic
   leukaemia), ulceration, infection,
   haemorrhage (marrow aplasia, etc.);
   atrophic glossitis, angular stomatitis
   (iron, vitamin deficiencies)
Tonsils—enlarged (lymphoma)

ARMS
Epitrochlear nodes (non-Hodgkin's
   lymphoma, chronic lymphocytic
   leukaemia, intravenous drug use,
   sarcoid)

LEGS
Vasculitis (Henoch-Schonlein purpura—
   buttocks, thighs)
Bruising
Pigmentation
Ulceration
Neurological signs (subacute combined
   degeneration, peripheral neuropathy)

OTHER
Fundi (hyperviscosity, haemorrhages,
   infection, etc.)
Temperature chart (infection)
Urine analysis (haematuria, bile, etc.)
Rectal examination (blood loss)
Hess Test

vasculitis. Pale palm creases may indicate anaemia (usually the haemoglobin level being lower than 90g/L). Evidence of arthropathy may be important, e.g., rheumatoid arthritis (p. 92) and Felty's syndrome, recurrent haemarthroses in bleeding disorders, secondary gout in myeloproliferative disorders (p. 84).

Examine the epitrochlear nodes. Do this by placing your palm under the patient's elbow—your thumb will be placed over the appropriate area (proximal and slightly anterior to the medial epicondyle). A palpable node is usually pathological and may indicate non-Hodgkin's lymphoma. Note any arm bruising. Remember petechiae are pinhead haemorrhages, while ecchymoses are larger bruises. Palpable purpura suggests vasculitis, dysglobulinaemia or bacteraemia.

Go to the axillae and palpate the axillary nodes. Do this by raising the patient's arm and placing your fingers as high as possible. Then position the patient's forearm comfortably over your own forearm. Use your left hand for the patient's right axilla and vice versa. There are 5 main areas: central; lateral (above and lateral); pectoral (most medial); subscapular (most inferior) and infraclavicular.

Look at the face. Inspecting the eyes, note jaundice, pallor or haemorrhage of the sclerae, or the injected sclera of polycythaemia. Examine the mouth. Note gum hypertrophy (differential diagnosis includes acute monocytic leukaemia and scurvy), ulceration, infection (e.g., moniliasis), haemorrhage, atrophic glossitis (secondary to iron, $B_{12}$ or folate deficiency) and angular stomatitis. Look for tonsillar and adenoid enlargement (Waldeyer's ring).

Sit the patient up. Examine the cervical nodes from behind. There are 7 groups: submental, submandibular, jugular chain, posterior triangle, postauricular, preauricular and occipital. Then feel the supraclavicular area from the front. Tap the spine with your fist for bony tenderness (which can be due to an enlarging marrow—e.g., in myeloma, carcinoma). Also gently press the sternum, clavicles and shoulders for bony tenderness.

Lie the patient flat again. Examine the abdomen (p. 165), particularly for splenomegaly (Table 8-19) and hepatomegaly (Tables 8-15 and 8-20). Don't forget to feel the testes, ask to do a rectal examination (for melaena or tumour) and spring the hips for pelvic tenderness. Palpate the inguinal nodes. There are 2 groups—along the inguinal ligament and along the femoral vessels.

Examine the legs. Note particularly leg ulcers which may occur with hereditary spherocytosis, sickle cell syndromes, thalassaemia, macroglobulinaemia, thrombotic thrombocytopenic purpura, polycythaemia and Felty's syndrome. Ask to examine the legs from a neurological aspect, for evidence of $B_{12}$ deficiency. Remember hypothyroidism and lead poisoning can cause anaemia and peripheral neuropathy. Do not miss Henoch-Schonlein purpura over the buttocks and legs.

Finally, ask to examine the fundi (engorged retinal vessels, papilloedema, haemorrhages, etc.) and look at the temperature chart. Also ask whether you can perform a Hess test if you suspect thrombocytopenia or capillary fragility. Be able to describe the Hess test—inflate the blood pressure cuff to 1.33kPa (10mmHg) above diastolic blood pressure. After 5 minutes, deflate the cuff then wait another 5 minutes and count the number of petechiae; more than 20/cm² is definitely abnormal. Causes of generalized lymphadenopathy are presented in Table 8-21.

**Table 8-21.** *Causes of Generalized Lymphadenopathy*

1. Lymphoma (rubbery and firm) (p. 87)
2. Leukaemia (chronic lymphocytic leukaemia, acute lymphoblastic leukaemia particularly)
3. Malignant disease (metastases or reactive changes causing usually asymmetrical very firm nodes)
4. Infections, e.g., viral (cytomegalovirus, HIV, infectious mononucleosis), bacterial (e.g., tuberculosis, brucellosis), protozoal (e.g., toxoplasmosis)
5. Connective tissue diseases, e.g., rheumatoid arthritis (p. 92), systemic plus erythematosus (p. 97)
6. Infiltrations, e.g., sarcoidosis (p. 58)
7. Drugs, e.g., phenytoin (pseudolymphoma)

# THE ENDOCRINE SYSTEM

## The Thyroid Gland

Please examine this patient's neck.

### *Method* (Figure 25)

The most likely problem is thyroid disease, but you should also consider in the neck examination the possibilities of superior vena caval obstruction (p. 159), cervical lymphadenopathy (p. 184), carotid aneurysm or bruit, jugular venous pressure abnormalities (p. 137) and tracheal deviation (p. 160).

Glance first at the face for signs of thyrotoxicosis and myxoedema (see below).

Inspect the neck for scars, swelling and prominent veins with the patient sitting up and the neck fully exposed. Look at the front and the sides. Next ask the patient to swallow a sip of water and look for thyroid enlargement, which moves up with swallowing.

First palpate gently from behind, with the neck flexed, feeling for any thyroid mass (Table 8-22). Note the shape, consistency and distribution of the thyroid enlargement. If a nodule is palpable, determine if this is single or part of a multinodular goiter. Ask the patient if the gland is tender (a clue to subacute thyroiditis) and note any hoarseness of the voice (due to recurrent laryngeal nerve palsy). Decide whether you can palpate the lower border of the gland (to exclude retrosternal extension) and whether there is a thrill. Feel for cervical lymphadenopathy from behind. Palpate each carotid artery (absence possibly indicating malignant infiltration). Test the sternomastoid function, as malignant disease may infiltrate this muscle. Finally, palpate the gland from in front and note the tracheal position.

Percuss over the upper part of the manubrium from one side to the other right across the bone and note any change from resonant to dull (a sign of retrosternal extension).

Auscultate over the thyroid gland for bruits (a sign of active thyrotoxicosis) and also over the carotid arteries.

Remember Pemberton's sign. Ask the patient to lift the arms over the head.

**Figure 25.**   *Neck*

Sitting up

GENERAL INSPECTION
   Face, e.g., thyrotoxicosis, myxoedema,
      other diagnostic facies (Table 8-29)

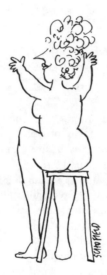

NECK
   Inspection
      Scars
      Swelling
      Prominent veins
      Swallowing (a glass of water)
   Palpation (from behind with neck flexed)
      Thyroid enlargement—note size,
      shape, consistency, borders,
      mobility
      Thyroid tenderness
      Thyroid thrill
      Cervical nodes
   Palpation (from in front)
      Thyroid (as above)
      Carotid arteries
      Supraclavicular nodes
      Trachea position
      Sternomastoid function
   Percuss
      Upper manubrium
   Auscultate
      Thyroid bruit
      Carotid bruit
   Pemberton's sign

OTHER
   Signs of thyrotoxicosis/myxoedema
      elsewhere
   Thyroidectomy scar—test for
      hypoparathyroidism
      (Chvostek's and Trousseau's signs)
   Jugular venous pressure, e.g.,
      superior vena cava obstruction
   Causes of localized cervical gland
      enlargement, e.g., chest, abdomen,
      head and neck examination

**Table 8-22.**  *Causes of a Diffuse Goitre*

1. Idiopathic (majority)
2. Puberty and pregnancy
3. Grave's disease
4. Thyroiditis: Hashimoto's thyroiditis; subacute thyroiditis (tender); chronic fibrosing (Reidel's) thyroiditis (rare)
5. Simple goitre (iodine deficiency)
6. Goitrogens, e.g., iodine excess, drugs (e.g., lithium, phenylbutazone)
7. Inborn errors of thyroid hormone synthesis, e.g., Pendred's syndrome, an autosomal recessive condition associated with nerve deafness

**Table 8-23.**  *Causes of Thyrotoxicosis*

**Primary:**
1. Grave's disease
2. Toxic adenoma or multinodular goitre
3. Hashimoto's thyroiditis (early in its course); subacute thyroiditis (transient)
4. Iodine-induced (after previous iodine deficiency)—termed the Jod-Basedow's phenomenon
5. Excess thyroid hormone replacement
6. Postpartum thyroiditis (non-tender)

**Secondary:**
1. Pituitary or ectopic thyroid stimulating hormone hypersecretion (very rare)
2. Hydatidiform mole or choriocarcinoma (HCG secretion—rare)
3. Struma ovarii (rare)
4. Factitious

N.B.  The 3 components of Graves' disease—viz., eye signs, hyperthyroidism with goitre and pretibial myxoedema—run independent courses. HCG = human chorionic gonadotrophin.

Look for suffusion of the face, elevation of the jugular venous pressure and inspiratory stridor. Any retrosternal mass may cause these changes.

If there is evidence of a goitre and obvious eye disease (indicating the presence of *thyrotoxicosis* [Table 8-23]), proceed to the face. Examine the eyes for exophthalmos by noting the presence of sclera below the cornea when she is looking straight ahead. Note lid retraction by looking for the presence of sclera above the cornea. Then test for lid lag by asking the patient to follow your finger descending at a moderate rate. Now examine the conjunctiva for chemosis. Test eye movements for ophthalmoplegia (p. 207). The inferior oblique muscle power is lost first, then convergence is affected, followed by the other muscles in thyrotoxicosis. Examine the fundi because optic atrophy can occur late. Then look from behind, over the patient's forehead, when she is looking forward, for proptosis.

Examine the outstretched hands for tremor. It is worthwhile placing a sheet of paper over the dorsal aspects of the fingers. Look at the nails for onycholysis (Plummer's nails)—distal separation of the nail from its bed—and thyroid acropachy (this looks like clubbing and is clubbing, but is not called clubbing). Note any palmar erythema. Feel for warmth and sweating. Feel the radial pulse for sinus tachycardia, atrial fibrillation or a collapsing pulse.

**Table 8-24.** *Causes of Hypothyroidism*

**Primary:**
*Without a goitre (decreased or absent thyroid tissue)*
Idiopathic atrophy
Treatment, e.g, I-131, surgery
Agenesis or a lingual thyroid
Unresponsiveness to thyroid stimulating hormone
*With a goitre (decreased synthesis)*
Chronic thyroiditis, e.g., late Hashimoto's disease, Reidel's
thyroiditis
Drugs, e.g., lithium, amiodarone
Endemic iodine deficiency
Iodine-induced hypothyroidism
Inborn errors (enzyme deficiency)
**Secondary:**
Pituitary lesions
**Tertiary:**
Hypothalamic lesions
**Transient:**
Thyroid hormone treatment withdrawn
Subacute thyroiditis
Postpartum thyroiditis

Test for proximal myopathy in the arms and tap the arm reflexes for briskness (p. 226).

If there is time, proceed to the legs and look for skin manifestations: pretibial myxoedema—bilateral firm, elevated dermal nodules and plaques which can be pink, brown, or skin coloured and caused by mucopolysaccharide accumulation—and vitiligo. Test for proximal myopathy and hyperreflexia in the legs.

Ask to examine the chest for evidence of gynaecomastia in men, and the heart for an ejection systolic murmur and signs of congestive cardiac failure. Although rarely of importance, there may also be signs of mild splenomegaly and hepatomegaly on abdominal examination, as well as generalized lymphadenopathy.

If a thyroidectomy scar is present, ask to look for the signs of hypocalcaemia, i.e., Chvostek's and Trousseau's signs. Chvostek's sign may be present in normal patients. It is tested by tapping over the facial nerve 3 to 5cm below and in front of the ear. The facial muscle twitches briefly in the presence of hypocalcaemia. Trousseau's sign is tested by pumping up a sphygmomanometer cuff above systolic blood pressure and looking for *main d' accoucheur* (a strongly adducted thumb with fingers extended except at the metacarpophalangeal joints) that occurs within 2 minutes.

If there is a suspicion of *hypothyroidism* (where goitre is unusual) (Table 8-24), proceed as follows. Examine the hands. Note peripheral cyanosis, swelling and dry, cold skin. Look at the palm creases for anaemia (Table 8-25). Feel the pulse

**Table 8-25.**  *Causes of Anaemia in Patients with Hypothyroidism*

1. Chronic disease (direct or erythropoietin-mediated depressive effect on bone marrow)
2. Folate deficiency secondary to bacterial overgrowth
3. Pernicious anaemia is associated with myxoedema
4. Iron deficiency in females due to menorrhagia
5. Haemolysis secondary to hypercholestrolaemia-induced spur-cell anaemia

for bradycardia and a small volume. Test for carpal tunnel syndrome by tapping over the flexor retinaculum medial to the base of the thenar eminence with the wrist extended. This sign (Tinel's) is positive if there is tingling over the median nerve distribution. Test for delayed relaxation of the biceps jerk.

Examine for proximal myopathy, which is rare, then proceed to the face. Note here any general swelling and periorbital oedema. Look for loss of the outer one-third of the eyebrows and periorbital xanthelasma. Note if the skin is dry, fine and smooth. There may be signs of carotenaemia, alopecia or vitiligo. Look at the tongue, which may be swollen, then ask the patient to tell you her name and address and note any hoarseness or slowness of speech. Test for nerve deafness, which may be bilateral.

Go to the legs next (p. 230). Examine them neurologically, starting with the ankle jerks, noting particularly any evidence of slow relaxation which is best seen with the patient kneeling on a chair. Then examine for peripheral neuropathy and look for other uncommon neurological abnormalities (Table 8-26).

Finally ask to examine the chest for pleural and pericardial effusions. There may be dry, rough 'sandpaper-like' skin over the chest.

# Panhypopituitarism

This man has lost his libido. Please assess him.

## *Method*

You cleverly note that this man looks 'panhypopituitary' (Table 8-27). Proceed as follows. Ask him to stand and make sure he is fully uncovered. Note the pale skin and the lack of hair. The patient may have short stature (failure of growth hormone secretion before growth is complete) and no secondary sexual characteristics (gonadotrophin failure before puberty).

Look at the face more closely. Multiple fine skin wrinkles around the eyes and mouth are characteristic of gonadotrophin deficiency. Look closely for a hypophy-sectomy scar on the forehead near the inner canthus of the eye. Examine the eyes (visual fields, especially for bitemporal hemianopia, fundi for optic atrophy) and assess cranial nerves III, IV, VI as well as the first division of V (affected by tumour extension into the cavernous sinus) (p. 205). Feel the facial hair over the beard area in men.

Go to the chest and look for decreased body hair, pale skin and gynaecomastia.

**Table 8-26.** *Neurological Associations of Hypothyroidism*

**Common:**
- 1. Entrapment, e.g., carpal tunnel, tarsal tunnel
- 2. Delayed relaxation phase of ankle jerks
- 3. Nerve deafness

**Uncommon:**
- 1. Peripheral neuropathy
- 2. Proximal myopathy (with normal creatinine kinase levels)
- 3. Hypokalemic periodic paralysis
- 4. Eaton-Lambert syndrome, deterioration or unmasking of myasthenia gravis
- 5. Cerebellar syndrome
- 6. Psychosis
- 7. Coma
- 8. Cerebrovascular disease
- 9. High cerebrospinal fluid protein
- 10. Muscle cramps

**Table 8-27.** *Causes of Panhypopituitarism*

1. Chromophobe adenoma (commonest cause in males)
2. Other space-occupying lesion (craniopharyngioma, metastatic carcinoma, granuloma)
3. Iatrogenic (surgery, radiation)
4. Sheehan's syndrome (post-partum necrosis)
5. Head injury
6. Idiopathic

N.B. Loss of function (in order)
60% pituitary loss: growth hormone, FSH, and LH
80% pituitary loss: TSH
100% pituitary loss: ACTH

FSH = follicle stimulating hormone; LH = luteinizing hormone; ACTH = adrenocorticotrophin; TSH = thyroid stimulating hormone

Lie the patient down and look for loss of pubic hair and testicular atrophy (testes small and firm—the normal size is 15 to 25mL in volume).

Test the ankle jerks (for hypothyroidism—there is no myxoedematous appearance) and ask to check the blood pressure lying and standing (hypotension with ACTH deficiency).

## Cushing's Syndrome

This patient has noted weight gain. Please make an examination.

### *Method* (Figure 26)

This type of introduction may mean Cushing's syndrome in the clinical examination. Make sure the patient is undressed to the underpants and standing. Look at the patient from the front, sides and behind.

Note central obesity, with peripheral sparing, and the skin for bruising, atrophy

**Figure 26.**  *Cushing's Syndrome*

Standing                                                    Sitting

GENERAL INSPECTION                                          FACE
   Central obesity and thin limbs                 Plethora, hirsutism, acne, telangiectasia
   Skin bruising, atrophy                           Moon shape
   Pigmentation (ACTH tumour—rare—                  Eyes—visual fields (pituitary
     or bilateral adrenalectomy)                tumour), fundi (atrophy, papilloedema,
   Poor wound healing                                 signs of hypertension or diabetes)
                                     Mouth—thrush
                                     Neck—supraclavicular fat pads

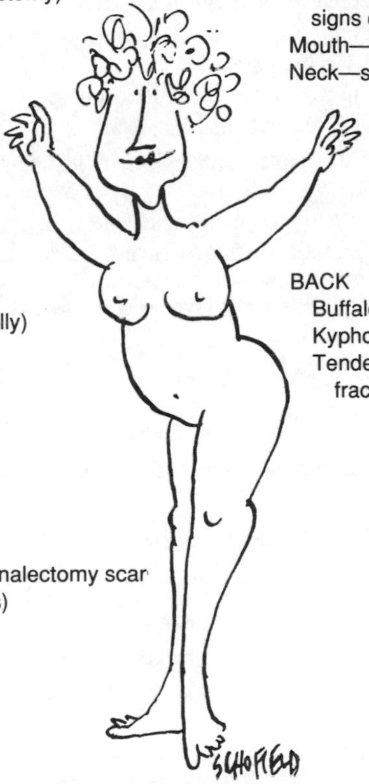

ARMS                                                        BACK
   Purple striae (proximally)                       Buffalo hump (interscapular fat pad)
   Proximal myopathy                                Kyphoscoliosis (osteoporosis)
                                     Tenderness of vertebrae (osteoporotic
                                       fractures)

Lying flat

ABDOMEN                                                     LEGS
   Purple striae                                    Squat (proximal myopathy)
   Adrenal masses, adrenalectomy scar               Striae (thighs)
   Liver (tumour deposits)                          Bruising, oedema

                                     MENTAL STATE
                                     Depression
                                     Psychosis
                                     Irritability

               OTHER
                 Urine analysis (glycosuria,
                    evidence of renal stone disease)
                 Blood pressure (hypertension)
                 Signs of ectopic tumour
                    (e.g., lung small cell carcinoma
                    or carcinoid)—rare

and pigmentation of extensor areas. Hyperpigmentation suggests an ectopic ACTH secreting tumour, or it may indicate an ACTH secreting pituitary adenoma in a patient who has had a bilateral adrenalectomy (Nelson's syndrome).

Test for proximal myopathy of the arms and also of the legs (by getting the patient to squat). Examine the back for a buffalo hump and feel it. Look for kyphoscoliosis and tap the spine for bony tenderness due to osteoporotic vertebral crush fractures.

Then sit the patient on the side of the bed. Look at the face for plethora, hirsutism, acne, telangiectasia and a moon shape.

Test the eyes for visual field defects and look in the fundi for papilloedema (due to benign intracranial hypertension or a pituitary tumour), optic atrophy, as well as hypertensive or diabetic changes (Tables 8-7, p. 158, 8-37, p. 200). Then look at the neck for supra-clavicular fat pads.

Ask the patient to lie down. Examine the abdomen (p. 165) for adrenalectomy scars, pigmentation, striae and adrenal masses. Look at the genitalia. Virilization in females or gynaecomastia in males suggests adrenal carcinoma is more likely. Next look at the legs for oedema, bruising and poor wound healing.

Don't forget to ask for the results of urine analysis (glucose) and take the blood pressure (hypertension). Diagnostic tests are summarized in Table 8-28.

## Acromegaly

This patient has noted some change in facial appearance. Please examine.

### Method (Figure 27)

Consider the possible diagnostic facies (Table 8-29). If the patient looks acromegalic, proceed as follows.

Have the patient stand, or sit on the side of the bed. Look at the hands. Look for the coarse features and spade-like shape as well as increased sweating and warmth. Tap over the flexor retinaculum for Tinel's sign. Feel the ulnar nerve for thickening at the elbow. Go to the arms and test for proximal myopathy. Also look in the axillae for skin tags (molluscum fibrosum), greasy skin and acanthosis nigricans (brown to back velvety elevation of the epidermis due to multiple confluent papillomas).

Go on to the face. Look for frontal bossing due to a large supraorbital ridge (which may also occur in rickets, Paget's disease, hydrocephalus or achondroplasia). Note if there is a large tongue (sometimes too big to fit into the mouth neatly). Enlargement of the lower jaw (called prognathism) and splaying of the teeth may be present. Notice any acne or hirsutism in women (Table 8-38, p. 201), and test the voice which may be deep, husky and resonant.

The eyes must be carefully examined. Visual fields should be checked—look particularly for bitemporal hemianopia, which is the classical sign but is uncommon; many field defects are possible (p. 213). Examine the fundi for optic atrophy, papilloedema and angioid streaks (red, brown or grey streaks 3 to 5 times the diameter of the retinal vein appearing to emanate form the optic disc and due to

**Table 8-28.**   *Diagnosis of Cushing's Syndrome*

(N.B. Cushing's disease is specifically pituitary ACTH overproduction.)

**Screening Tests**

1. Cortisol levels morning and evening: loss of diurnal rhythm (evening cortisol level should be less than half the morning value) of little diagnostic value.

2. 24-hour urine collection for urinary free cortisol determination (an indirect assessment of cortisol production).

3. Overnight dexamethasone suppression test (1mg dexamethasone at midnight causes suppression of cortisol in normal subjects at 9:00 a.m.). No suppression is found in Cushing's syndrome, but this may also occur with alcoholism, induction of hepatic enzymes (e.g., phenytoin), depression, in patients taking the contraceptive pill and in some obese patients.

4. Blood count (secondary polycythaemia, neutrophil leukocytosis, eosinopenia).

5. Electrolyte levels (hypokalaemic alkalosis, particularly with ectopic ACTH-producing tumours).

6. Blood sugar level (hyperglycaemia).

**Definitive Tests**

1. 2mg dexamethasone suppression test (0.5mg sixth hourly for 48 hours). No suppression of plasma cortisol or urinary free cortisol occurs in Cushing's syndrome, but usually suppression does occur in normal subjects, obese patients and depressed patients.

2. 8mg dexamethasone suppression test (2mg sixth hourly for 48 hours). Suppression occurs in Cushing's disease, but no suppression is usually found in adrenal adenoma or carcinoma or in the presence of ectopic ACTH production. False-positive results can occur in patients taking anticonvulsants (which accelerate dexamethasone metabolism).

3. Metapyrone test—this drug inhibits 11 beta-hydroxylase; 3g can be given at midnight. Early morning plasma 11-deoxycortisol and urinary 17-hydroxycorticoid or ketogenic steroids increase in Cushing's disease but not in other causes of Cushing's syndrome. If the results of the high-dose dexamethasome suppression and metapyrone tests are discordant, ectopic ACTH secretion should be strongly suspected.

4. Corticotropin-releasing hormone (CRH) stimulation test—CRH stimulates the release of ACTH normally; in Cushing's disease an intravenous injection of ovine CRH increases plasma ACTH, but this does not occur with ectopic ACTH production or adrenal neoplasms.

5. ACTH level—high in ectopic ACTH production, low with adrenal adenoma or carcinoma, high or normal in Cushing's disease. Ectopic secretion of CRH by tumours is a very rare cause of Cushing's syndrome.

6. Petrosal sinus ACTH sampling—a central to peripheral venous cortisol ratio of >2:1 is diagnostic of Cushing's disease; lateralization of ACTH production helps the neurosurgeon plan transsphenoidal exploration of the sella.

N.B.  If Cushing's disease is present, pituitary assessment is necessary. If adrenal disease is suspected, CT scan is useful to assess the anatomy. Remember ectopic ACTH production by a tumour (e.g., small cell carcinoma of lung, carcinoid of lung or thymus, pancreatic islet cell carcinoma, ovarian carcinoma) does not usually cause Cushingoid clinical features but may present with hyperpigmentation and hypokalaemic alkalosis.

**Figure 27.**   *Acromegaly Examination*

GENERAL INSPECTION                          FACE
  Diagnostic facies                           Frontal bossing
                                              Hirsutism
                                              Macroglossia
HANDS                                         Prognathism
  Shape                                       Hoarseness
  Sweat
  Tinel's sign (carpal tunnel)

                                            EYES
ULNA NERVE                                    Visual fields
  Thickened                                   Cranial nerves III, IV
                                              VI, V
                                              Fundi
PROXIMAL MYOPATHY

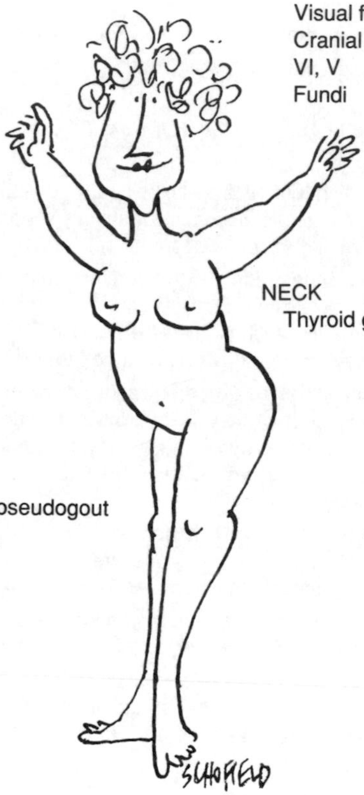

HEART
  Cardiac failure

                                            NECK
                                              Thyroid gland (diffuse or nodular goitre)

ABDOMEN
  Organomegaly

LOWER LIMBS
  Hips   } osteoarthritis, pseudogout
  Knees                                     AXILLAE
  Entrapment neuropathy                       Skin tags
  Heel pad thickening                         Acanthosis nigricans
                                              Greasy skin

OTHER
  Urine analysis (glycosuria)
  Rectal examination—colonic polyps
    (correlate with skin tags)
  Blood pressure (hypertension)
  Sleep apnoea

**Table 8-29.** *Common Diagnostic Facies*

 1. Acromegalic
 2. Thyrotoxic (p. 187)
 3. Myxoedematous (p. 188)
 4. Cushingoid (p. 190)
 5. Pagetic (p. 105)
 6. Myotonic (p. 244)
 7. Parkinsonian (p. 249)
 8. Thalassaemia (p. 81)
 9. Marfanoid (p. 158)
10. Mitral (p. 137)

degeneration of Bruch's membrane with resultant fibrosis [Table 8-30]). There may also be diabetic (p. 200) or hypertensive changes (p. 158).

Examine the thyroid gland for diffuse enlargement or a multinodular goitre (p. 185).

Ask next whether you may examine the cardiovascular system for signs of congestive cardiac failure, the abdomen for organomegaly—of liver, spleen and kidney—and for signs of hypogonadism (secondary to an enlarging pituitary adenoma). Ask to examine the lower limbs for osteoarthritis and pseudogout. Also, if allowed, look for foot drop (entrapment of common peroneal nerve) and heel pad thickening.

If there is time look for evidence of hypothyroidism and adrenocortical insufficiency (from an enlarging pituitary adenoma).

Don't forget to ask for the results of urine analysis to exclude glycosuria secondary to glucose intolerance, and take the blood pressure (hypertension is an association). Decide if the acromegaly is active (Table 8-31). Ask if any photographs taken of the patient over the years are available for inspection (typically manifestations begin in middle age). Diagnostic tests are summarized in Table 8-32.

## Addison's Disease

This patient has weakness, anorexia and weight loss. Please assess.

### *Method*

Fortunately you suspect Addison's disease. Undress the patient and look for pigmentation (particularly in the palm creases, elbows, gums and buccal mucosa, genital areas and scars) and vitiligo, due to an autoimmune disease association. Ear lobe calcification occurs rarely.

Take the blood pressure and test for a postural drop. Ask for the results of a urine analysis, as diabetes is associated with Addison's disease. Remember the rest of the autoimmune cluster may also be associated (Table 8-33) and the possible causes (Table 8-34). Diagnostic tests are summarized in Table 8-35.

**Table 8-30.**   *Causes of Angioid Streaks (mnemonic PASH)*

1. P Paget's disease; Pseudoxanthoma elasticum; Poisoning (lead)
2. A Acromegaly
3. S Sickle cell anaemia
4. H Hyperphosphataemia (familial)

**Table 8-31.**   *Evidence of Activity in Acromegaly*

1. Skin tag number
2. Excessive sweating
3. Presence of glycosuria
4. Increasing visual field loss or development of cranial nerve palsies of III, IV, VI and V
5. Enlarging goitre
6. Hypertension
7. Symptoms of headache, or increasing ring size, shoe size or denture size.

**Table 8-32.**   *The Diagnosis of Acromegaly*

**Anatomical (99% pituitary adenoma)**
   Skull X-ray film (enlarged sella, double floor)
   CT or MRI scan
**Biochemical:**
   Insulin-like growth factor (IGF)-1 (Somatomedin C) level in plasma (elevated in active
      acromegaly)
   Glucose tolerance test (no suppression or a paradoxical rise in growth hormone level)
   Thyrotropin-releasing hormone test (abnormal release of growth hormone in 80%).
   Evaluate pituitary function—static and dynamic tests

**Table 8-33.**   *Autoimmune-associated Disease*

Addison's Disease
Hypoparathyroidism
Mucocutaneous Candidiasis
Diabetes Mellitus (type I)
Hashimoto's Thyroiditis
Grave's Disease
Primary Ovarian Failure
Pernicious Anaemia
Vitiligo

**Table 8-34.** *Causes of Addison's Disease (Chronic Adrenal Insufficiency)\**

**Primary**

Autoimmune adrenal disease (>80% of all cases)

Polyglandular syndromes:

*Type I:* Addison's disease, hypoparathyroidism and mucocutaneous candidiasis (anti-IgA antibodies)

*Type II:* Addison's disease, type I diabetes mellitus and Hashimoto's thyroiditis or Grave's disease

Tuberculosis, histoplasmosis

Infiltration, e.g., amyloidosis, sarcoidosis

Metastatic malignant disease

Demyelinating disease: adrenoleukodystrophy (asymmetrical cortical signs and Addison's disease), adrenomyeloneuropathy (spastic paraparesis and Addison's disease)

Drugs, e.g., heparin (bilateral adrenal haemorrhage), aminoglutethamide, ketoconazole HIV infection

**Secondary**

Pituitary or hypothalamic disease (usually *no* mineralocorticoid deficiency)

\* N.B. Acute adrenal insufficiency may follow any stress in a patient with chronic hypoadrenalism or abrupt cessation of prolonged high-dose steroid therapy.

**Table 8-35.** *Diagnosis of Addison's Disease*

**Screening Tests:**

Electrolyte levels (hyponatraemia, hyperkalaemia, hyperchloraemic acidosis, hypercalcaemia)
Hypoglycaemia
Blood count (lymphocytosis, eosinophilia)
Chest X-ray film (tuberculosis, small heart)
Plain abdominal X-ray film (adrenal calcification)

**Definitive Tests:**

Short Synacthen test (0.25mg synthetic ACTH given intramuscularly)
Long Synacthen test (8-hour intravenous infusion or depot administration) if subnormal response
Plasma ACTH level

# Diabetes Mellitus

Please examine this diabetic patient.

## *Method* (Figure 28)

General inspection may reveal a characteristic facial appearance (e.g., Cushing's syndrome or acromegaly) or pigmentation (e.g., haemochromatosis) which will modify the examination approach. Otherwise, expose the patient's legs. This is the only case in which there is an advantage in starting at the legs.

**Figure 28.** *Diabetes Mellitus*

Lying

GENERAL INSPECTION
Weight—obesity
Hydration
Endocrine facies (Table 8-29)
Pigmentation—
    haemochromatosis, etc.

EYES
Fundi—cataracts, rubeosis, retinal
    disease
III nerve palsy, etc.

MOUTH AND EARS
Infection

NECK
Carotid arteries—palpate, auscultate

CHEST
Signs of infection

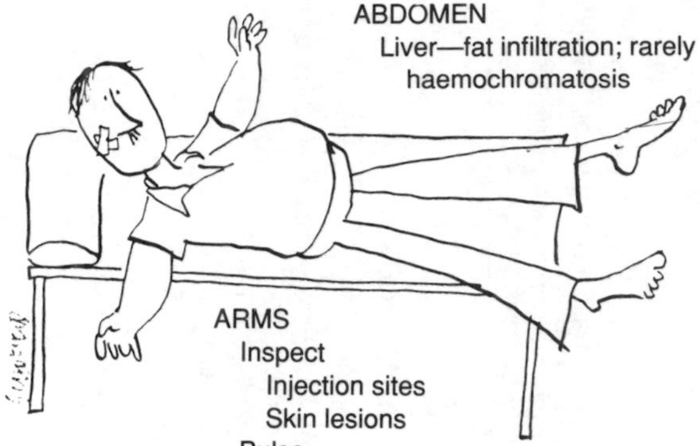

ABDOMEN
Liver—fat infiltration; rarely
    haemochromatosis

ARMS
Inspect
    Injection sites
    Skin lesions
Pulse

OTHER
Urine analysis—glycosuria, ketones,
    proteinuria
Blood pressure and pulse—
    lying and standing

LEGS
Inspect
    Skin—necrobiosis, hair loss,
        infection, pigmented scars, atrophy,
        ulceration, injection sites
    Muscle wasting
Palpate
    Temperature feet (cold, blue
        due to small or large vessel
        disease)
Peripheral pulses
    Femoral (auscultate)
    Popliteal
    Posterior tibial
    Dorsalis pedis
Oedema
Neurological assessment
    Femoral nerve mononeuritis
    Peripheral neuropathy

**Table 8-36.** *Autonomic Neuropathy*

**Clinical features:**
Postural hypotension [a blood pressure fall of >4/2.67kpa (>30/20mmHg) on standing upright
    from a supine position]
Loss of sinus arrhythmia
Loss of sweating
Impotence
Nocturnal diarrhoea
Urine retention, incontinence
Valsalva manoeuvre causes no slowing of the pulse

Look for necrobiosis lipodica over the shins (a central yellow scarred area with a surrounding red margin if active, due to atrophy of subcutaneous collagen—it is rare), pigmented scars, skin atrophy, small rounded plaques with raised borders lying in a linear fashion over the shins (diabetic dermopathy), ulceration and infection. Look at the thigh for injection sites, fat atrophy or fat hypertrophy due to impure insulin use, and quadriceps wasting, from femoral nerve mononeuritis—called (inaccurately) diabetic amyotrophy.

Look for loss of hair, skin atrophy and blue cool feet (small vessel vascular disease). Feel all the peripheral pulses and note capillary return. Feel for pitting oedema. Auscultate over the femoral artery for bruits.

Test proximal muscle power and test the reflexes. Assess for peripheral neuropathy, including dorsal column loss—called diabetic pseudotabes (p. 242). Charcot's joints (due to proprioceptive loss) may rarely be present.

Go to the upper limbs. Look at the nails for candida infection. Feel the upper arm injection sites. Ask for the blood pressure lying and standing to detect autonomic neuropathy (Table 8-36).

Now examine the eyes for visual acuity. Remember episodes of poor control cause lens abnormalities acutely. Look for Argyll Robertson pupils (which are rare). Remember a diabetic third nerve palsy is usually pupil sparing—infarction affects the inner more than the outer fibres, while compressive lesions affect the outer fibres first and so involve the pupil early. Look in the fundi (Table 8-37). Whilst performing fundoscopy also note the presence of cataracts and any new blood vessel formation over the iris (rubeosis). Always test the III, IV and VI cranial nerves and remember other cranial nerves may also be affected (p. 205). Periorbital and perinasal swelling with gangrene can occur with rhinocerebral mucormycosis, an opportunistic fungal infection. Look in the mouth for monilia and other infection. Look in the ears for infection (e.g., malignant otitis externa due to *Pseudomonas aeruginosa*). Feel and auscultate the carotid arteries.

Ask to examine for hepatomegaly due to fatty infiltration and then ask for results of urine analysis with respect to glucose and protein. There may be signs of chronic renal failure with advanced disease (p. 113). Ask whether you may weigh the patient.

**Table 8-37.**  *Features of Diabetic Retinopathy*

**Non-Proliferative**
Haemorrhages:
1. Dot-haemorrhage into the inner retinal areas
2. Blot-haemorrhage into more superficial nerve fibre layers

Hard exudate (have straight edges)—leakage of protein and lipids from damaged capillaries
Soft exudate (cotton wool spots): have a fluffy appearance due to microinfarcts
Microaneurysms
Dilated veins

**Proliferative**
New vessels
Vitreous haemorrhage
Scar formation
Retinal detachment (opalescent sheet which balloons forward into the vitreous)
Laser scars (small brown or yellow spots)

## Hirsutism

A diagnostic approach is summarized in Table 8-38.

# THE RHEUMATOLOGICAL SYSTEM

In this section only the common joints which are encountered in the examination will be discussed.

## The Hands

Please examine this patient's hands.

### *Method* (Figure 29)

When you are asked to examine the hands consider the possibilities of arthropathy, acromegaly (p. 192), a peripheral nerve lesion (p. 236), a myopathy (p. 243) or a neuropathy (p. 234). If there is obvious joint disease, examine as follows.

First put the patient's hands on a pillow, palms down. You may ask the examiner if he or she minds whether you talk as you go. If he or she does not object, we believe this is the best way to proceed with a joint examination. However, also practise examining this sort of case by presenting at the end of the examination.

If the patient has arthropathy with an obvious rheumatoid distribution, start by stating that the patient has a symmetrical deforming polyarthropathy involving the wrists and hands. Then describe the wrists—look at the skin for erythema, atrophy, scars and rashes (e.g., psoriasis). Then look for swelling and its distribution, wrist deformity and muscle wasting.

Go on to the metacarpophalangeal joints. Mention, if present, any skin abnormalities, swelling and deformity, particularly ulnar deviation and volar subluxation.

**Table 8-38.** *Hirsutism*

*Clinical approach:*
General appearance [e.g., acromegaly (p. 192), Cushingoid (p. 190)]
Skin changes of porphyria cutanea tarda

*Hair distribution:*
Face
Midline (front and back)
Genital

*Signs of virilization:*
Receding hairline and increased oiliness of skin
Breast atrophy
Muscle bulk
Clitoromegaly

*Abdomen:*
Adrenal masses (rarely palpable)
Polycystic ovaries or ovarian tumour (rarely palpable)

*Blood pressure:*
Raised in C-11 hydroxylase deficiency

Causes of hirsutism:
1. Constitutional (normal endocrinology)
2. Polycystic ovaries, ovarian tumour, Idiopathic ovarian disease
3. Adrenal (e.g., Cushing's syndrome, congenital adrenal hyperplasia [21- or 11-hydroxylase deficiency], virilizing adrenal tumour)
4. Ovary (e.g., tumour)
5. Drugs (e.g., phenytoin, diazoxide, streptomycin, minoxidil, androgen, glucocorticoids)
6. Other (e.g., acromegaly, porphyria cutanea tarda)

Next describe the proximal and distal interphalangeal joints. Again mention any skin changes that may be present, swelling over each joint if present, and deformity, particularly 'swan necking' and *boutonniére* deformity of the fingers and 'Z' deformity of the thumb. Sausage-shaped phalanges occur in psoriatic arthropathy as well as ankylosing spondylitis and Reiter's disease.

Next look at the nails and describe any psoriatic nail changes, namely pitting, onycholysis, hyperkeratosis, ridging and discoloration. Note the signs of vasculitis (splinter haemorrhages, or black to brown 1 to 2mm skin infarcts usually in a periungual location) and mention this to the examiners.

Next turn the wrists over and look at the palms for scars, palmar erythema and muscle wasting.

Now go on and palpate each joint, starting with the wrists. Feel for synovitis (boggy swelling) and effusions. Describe the range of passive movement of the joint. Also note any joint crepitus. Palpate the ulnar styloid for tenderness. When examining the metacarpophalangeal joints also feel for subluxation. Test for palmar tendon crepitus (tenosynovitis).

Having examined each joint, assess the function of the hand. This is very important. Test grip strength, key grip and opposition strength (thumb and little finger), and ask the patient to perform a practical procedure like undoing a button.

**Figure 29.**  *Hands*

Sitting up (hands on a pillow)

GENERAL INSPECTION
  Cushingoid
  Weight
  Iritis, scleritis, etc.
  Obvious other joint disease

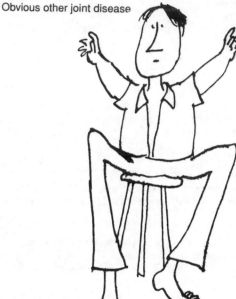

LOOK
  Dorsal aspect
    Wrists
      Skin—scars, redness, atrophy, rash
      Swelling—distribution
      Deformity
      Muscle wasting
    Metacarpophalangeal Joints
      Skin
      Swelling—distribution
      Deformity—ulnar deviation, volar
    subluxation, etc.
      Proximal and distal interphalangeal
      joints
    Skin
    Swelling—distribution
    Deformity—swan necking, *Boutonniere*,
      Z, sausage-shaped, etc.
    Nails
      Psoriatic changes—pitting, ridging,
    onycholysis, hyperkeratosis,
    discolouration

  Palmar aspect
    Skin—scars, palmar erythema, palm
      creases (anaemia), discolouration
    Muscle wasting

FEEL AND MOVE PASSIVELY
  Wrists
    Synovitis
    Effusions
    Range of movement
    Crepitus
    Ulnar styloid tenderness
  Metacarpophalangeal joints
    Synovitis
    Effusions
    Range of movement
    Crepitus
    Subluxation
  Proximal and distal interphalangeal joints
    As above
  Palmar tendon crepitus
  Carpal tunnel syndrome tests

HAND FUNCTION
  Grip strength
  Key grip
  Opposition strength
  Practical ability

OTHER
  Elbows—subcutaneous nodules, psoriatic
    rash
  Other joints
  Signs of systemic disease

**Table 8-39.** *The Seronegative Spondyloarthropathies*

|  | HLA B27 |
| --- | --- |
| 1. Ankylosing spondylitis | 95% |
| 2. Psoriatic spondylitis | 50% |
| 3. Reactive arthritis including Reiter's syndrome | 80% |
| 4. Enteropathic arthritis | 75% |

A formal neurological examination is not required in assessing arthropathy. Taping over the flexor retinaculum (Tinel's sign) may demonstrate median nerve entrapment (p. 237). After you have finished with the hands, feel at the elbows for rheumatoid nodules and look carefully for any psoriatic rash there also.

You should now have an idea of the pattern and severity of the deformity as well as the extent of the loss of function, and the activity of the disease.

Always consider the differential diagnosis of a deforming polyarthropathy:

1. Rheumatoid arthritis (p. 92).
2. Seronegative arthropathies—particularly psoriatic arthritis.
3. Polyarticular gout or pseudogout.
4. Primary generalized osteoarthritis (where distal and proximal interphalangeal joint involvement is common).

Look carefully while doing your hand examination for any of these possibilities.

At the end ask whether you may examine all the other joints which are likely to be involved and also other systems which are likely to be affected (p. 92).

## The Knees

Examine this patient's knees.

### *Method*

Expose both knees and thighs fully and have the patient lie on his or her back.

Look for quadriceps wasting and then over the knees for any skin abnormalities (scars or rashes), swelling and deformity. Synovial swelling is seen medial to the patella and in the suprapatella area. Fixed flexion deformity must be assessed. This is looked for here by inspecting the knee from the side (a space beneath the knee is seen).

Feel the quadriceps for wasting. Ask about tenderness and palpate for warmth and synovitis over the knee joint. Examine for effusions—the patella tap (ballottement) is used to confirm a large effusion. Here the fluid from the suprapatellar bursa is pushed by your hand into the joint space by squeezing the lower part of the quadriceps and then the patella is pushed downwards with the fingers. The patella will be ballotable if fluid is present under the patella.

Test flexion and extension passively and note the range of movement and the presence or absence of crepitus. Now examine for fixed flexion deformity by gently extending the knee. Test the ligaments next. The lateral and medial collateral ligaments are tested by having the knee slightly flexed, holding the leg with the right hand and arm, steadying the thigh with the left hand and moving the leg laterally and medially. Movements of more than 5 to 10 degrees are abnormal. The cruciate ligaments are tested by steadying the foot with your elbow and moving the leg anteriorly and posteriorly with the other hand. Again, laxity of more than 5 to 10 degrees is abnormal.

Finally, ask the patient to stand up and examine for a Baker's cyst, which is felt in the popliteal fossa and is more obvious when the knee is extended.

Proceed then to examine other joints that may be involved.

## The Feet

Examine this patient's feet.

### Method

Start by inspecting the ankles. Look at the skin (for scars and rashes) and look for swelling, deformity and muscle wasting. Examine the midfoot and forefoot similarly. Deformities affecting the forefoot include hallux valgus and clawing and crowding of the toes (in rheumatoid arthritis). Note any psoriatic nail changes. Look at the transverse and longitudinal arches. Look for callus over the metatarsal heads which occurs in subluxation.

Palpate, starting with the ankle, feeling for synovitis and effusion. Passive movement of the talar joints (dorsiflexion and plantar flexion) and subtalar joints (inversion and eversion) must be assessed. Tenderness on movement is more important than range of movement. The midfoot (midtarsal joint) allows rotation of the forefoot on a fixed hindfoot. Squeeze the metatarsophalangeal joints for tenderness. Examining the individual toes is useful in seronegative spondyloarthropathies and psoriatic arthritis where a sausage-like swelling of the toe is characteristic of these conditions.

Finally feel the Achilles tendon for nodules and palpate the inferior aspect of the heel for tenderness (plantar fasciitis).

Go on to examine other joints as is appropriate.

## The Back

Examine this patient's back.

### Method

The patient will commonly have ankylosing spondylitis (Table 8-39). Ask the patient to undress to the underpants and stand up. Look for deformity, inspecting from both the back and the side, particularly for loss of kyphosis and lumbar lordosis. Palpate each vertebral body for tenderness and palpate for muscle spasm.

Test movement next. Measure the finger–floor distance (inability to touch the toes suggests early lumbar disease). Next look at extension, lateral flexion and rotation of the back. Ask whether you may perform a modified Schober's test.

**Table 8-40.**  *The Cauda Equina Syndrome*

Back, buttock and leg pain
Lower limb weakness
Loss of sphincter control
Saddle sensory loss

**Table 8-41.**  *X-ray Changes in Ankylosing Spondylitis*

**Sacroiliac joints:**
1. Cortical outline lost (early)
2. Juxta-articular osteosclerosis
3. Erosions
4. Joint obliteration

**Lumbar spine:**
1. Loss of lumbar lordosis
2. Squaring of vertebrae
3. Syndesmophytes (thoracolumbar region)
4. Bamboo spine (bony bridging of vertebrae) and osteoporosis
5. Apophyseal joint fusion

This involves identifying the level of the posterior iliac spine on the vertebral body (approximately at L5). Place a mark 5cm below this point and another 10cm above this point. The patient is asked to touch his toes. There should normally be an increase of 5cm or more in the distance between the marks. In ankylosing spondylitis there will be little separation of the marks as all the movement is taking place at the hips. Next test the occiput to wall distance; have the patient place the heels and back against the wall and to touch the wall with the back of the head without raising the chin above the carrying level; inability to touch the wall suggests cervical involvement, and the distance from occiput to wall is measured.

Ask the patient to go back to bed and lie on his or her stomach.

A simple (and unreliable) test for sacroiliac disease is to push with the heel of the hand on the sacrum and note the presence of tenderness in either sacroiliac joint on springing (N.B. usually there is bilateral disease in ankylosing spondylitis).

Go to the heels and examine for Achilles tendonitis and plantar fasciitis which are characteristic of the spondyloarthropathies.

Ask next whether you can examine the chest for decreased lung expansion (chest expansion of less than 5cm at the nipple line suggests early costovertebral involvement) and apical fibrosis (p. 160). Ask whether you may also examine the heart, for aortic incompetence, mitral valve prolapse and evidence of conduction defects (p. 135), the eyes for uveitis, and the other large joints, particularly knees, hips and shoulders.

Rarely patients with ankylosing spondylitis have a cauda equina compression (see Table 8-40). Ask whether you may examine the rectum and stool for evidence of inflammatory bowel disease (p. 68), and for signs of amyloid deposition (e.g., hepatosplenomegaly, abnormal urine analysis results). Remember also to check for signs of psoriasis and Reiter's syndrome, which may cause spondylitis and unilateral sacroiliitis. X-ray changes are described in Table 8-41.

# THE NERVOUS SYSTEM

## Cranial Nerves

Examine this patient's cranial nerves.

### *Method*

Inspect the head and neck briefly first. Have the patient sit over the edge of the bed facing you and look for any craniotomy scars (often well disguised by hair), neurofibromata, hydrocephalus, Cushing's syndrome, acromegaly, Paget's disease, facial asymmetry and obvious ptosis, proptosis, skew deviation of the eyes or pupil inequality.

### *First Nerve* (p. 211)

Ask the examiners if they want you to test smell. They will rarely allow you to proceed as it is time consuming and not usually fruitful in examinations. If you are required to test smell, a series of sample bottles will be provided by the examiners containing vanilla, coffee, or other non-pungent substances. Remember to test each nostril separately (p. 211 for the causes of anosmia).

### *Second Nerve* (p. 211)

Test visual acuity (with the patient's spectacles on if he uses them for reading, as refractive errors are not cranial nerve abnormalities) using a visual acuity chart (p. 27). Test each eye separately, covering the other eye with a small card.

Examine the visual fields by confrontation using a red-tipped hat pin making sure your head is level with the patient's head. A red pin enables you to detect earlier peripheral field loss. Test each eye separately. If the patient has such poor acuity that a pin is difficult to use, map the fields with your fingers. When you are testing his right eye, he should look straight into your left eye. His head should be at arm's length and the patient should cover the eye not being tested with his hand. Bring the pin from the four main directions diagonally towards the centre of the field of vision.

Next map out the blind spot by asking about disappearance of the pin lateral to the centre of the field of vision of each eye. A gross enlargement may be detectable by comparison with your own blind spot.

Look into the fundi (p. 209).

### *Third, Fourth, and Sixth Nerves* (p. 215)

Look at the pupils. Note the shape, relative sizes and any associated ptosis. Use your pocket torch and shine the light from the side to gauge the reaction to light on both sides. Don't bore the examiner by shining the light several times into each eye—practise assessing the direct and consensual responses rapidly.

Look for the Marcus Gunn phenomenon (Afferent Pupillary Defect) by moving the torch in an arc from pupil to pupil. The affected pupil will paradoxically dilate after a short time when the torch is moved from a normal eye to one with optic atrophy or very decreased visual acuity from other causes. Test accommodation by asking the patient to look into the distance and then at your red pin placed about 15cm from his nose.

Assess eye movements with both eyes first. Ask the patient to look voluntarily and then follow the red pin in each direction—right and left lateral gaze, plus up and down in the lateral position. Look for failure of movement and nystagmus. Ask about diplopia (double vision) when the eyes are in each position. With complex lesions then assess each eye separately. Move the patient's head if the patient is unable to follow movements. Beware of strabismus.

*Fifth Nerve* (p. 218)

Ask permission first to test the corneal reflexes. Make sure you touch the cornea (not the conjunctiva) gently with a piece of cotton wool. Come in from the side and do this only once on each side. If the nerve pathways are intact, the patient will blink both eyes. Ask him if he can actually feel the touch (V is the sensory component). N.B. With an ipsilateral VII palsy, only the contralateral eye will blink—sensation is preserved (VII is the motor component). Also with an ipsilateral VII palsy, the eye on the side of the lesion may roll superiorly with the corneal stimulus ('Bell's phenomenon').

Test facial sensation in the 3 divisions, ophthalmic, maxillary and mandibular. Use a pin first to assess pain. Map out any area of sensory loss from dull to sharp and check for any loss up on the posterior part of the head ($C_2$) and neck ($C_3$). Light touch must be tested also, as there may be some sensory dissociation. N.B. A medullary or upper cervical lesion of V causes loss of pain and temperature sensation with preservation of light touch. A pontine lesion may cause loss of light touch with preservation of pain and temperature sensation.

Examine the motor division by asking the patient to clench his teeth (feeling the masseter muscles) and open his mouth; the pterygoid muscles will not allow you to force it closed if the nerve is intact. A unilateral lesion causes the jaw to deviate towards the weak (affected) side.

Always test the jaw jerk (with the mouth just open, the finger over the jaw is tapped with a tendon hammer). An increased jaw jerk occurs in pseudobulbar palsy.

*Seventh Nerve* (p. 218)

Look for facial asymmetry and then test the muscles of facial expression. Ask the patient to look up and wrinkle his forehead. Look for loss of wrinkling and feel the muscle strength by pushing down on each side. This is preserved in an upper motor neurone lesion because of bilateral cortical representation of these muscles.

Next ask the patient to shut his eyes tight—compare how deeply the eye lashes are buried on the two sides and then try to open each eye. Tell him to grin and compare the nasolabial grooves.

If a lower motor neurone lesion is detected, quickly check for ear and palatal vesicles for herpes zoster of the geniculate ganglion—the Ramsay Hunt syndrome. Examining for taste on the anterior two-thirds of the tongue is not usually required.

### Eighth Nerve (p. 220)

Whisper softly a number two feet away from each ear and ask the patient to tell you the number. Perform Rinne's and Weber's tests with a 256 Hertz tuning fork (p. 220). If indicated, ask for an auroscope (wax is the commonest cause of conduction deafness).

### Ninth and Tenth Nerves (p. 220)

Look at the palate and note any uvular displacement. Ask the patient to say 'aaah' and look for asymmetrical movement of the soft palate. With a unilateral lesion the uvula is drawn towards the unaffected (normal) side.

Gently perform a gag reflex (IX is the sensory component and X the motor component); touch the back of the pharynx on each side. Remember to ask the patient if he feels the spatula each time. You may lose marks if the patient vomits all over your examiner.

Ask the patient to speak (to assess hoarseness) and to cough (listen for a bovine cough which may occur with a recurrent laryngeal nerve lesion). N.B. You will not usually be required to test taste on the posterior one-third of the tongue (i.e., IX nerve).

### Eleventh Nerve

Ask the patient to shrug his shoulders and then feel the trapezius bulk and push the shoulders down. Then instruct the patient to turn his head against resistance (your hand) and also feel the muscle bulk of the sternomastoids.

### Twelfth Nerve (p. 221)

Whilst examining at the mouth, inspect the tongue for wasting and fasciculation (best seen with the tongue not protruded and which may be unilateral or bilateral). Next ask the patient to protrude his tongue. With a unilateral lesion the tongue deviates towards the weaker (affected) side.

The way to finish your assessment depends entirely on your findings. For example, if you discover evidence for a particular syndrome (such as the lateral medullary syndrome p. 209), you should proceed to confirm your impressions by examining more peripherally, if allowed (especially for long tract signs). If you discovered multiple lower cranial nerve palsies, you would want to assess, among other things, the nasopharynx for signs of tumour.

Auscultating for carotid and cranial bruits (over the mastoids, temples and orbits) as well as taking the blood pressure and testing the urine for sugar, is often relevant.

# Eyes

Examine this patient's eyes.

## *Method* (Figure 30)

Always inspect first, with the patient sitting over the end of the bed facing you at eye level if possible.

First note any corneal abnormalities, e.g., band keratopathy (in hypercalcaemic states) or Kayser-Fleischer rings (Wilson's disease—Adelaide candidates beware). Look at the sclerae for colour (e.g., jaundice, blue in osteogenesis imperfecta), pallor, injection and telangiectasia. Inspect carefully for subtle ptosis.

Look for exophthalmos from behind and above the patient, as well as in front (p. 187).

Proceed then as for the cranial nerve eye examination, i.e., testing acuity, fields and pupils and then performing fundoscopy (p. 206).

Begin fundoscopy by examining the cornea and lens, and then the retina. Note any corneal, lens or humor abnormalities. Look for retinal changes of diabetes mellitus (Table 8-37) and hypertension (Table 8-7). Also carefully inspect for optic atrophy, papilloedema, angioid streaks (Table 8-30), retinal detachment, central vein or artery thrombosis and retinitis pigmentosa.

Test eye movements. Also look for fatiguability of eye muscles by asking your patient to look up at your pin for half a minute (myasthenia gravis—p. 124). Test for lid lag if you suspect hyperthyroidism.

Test the corneal reflex.

Palpate the orbits for tenderness and auscultate the eyes with the bell of the stethoscope (the eye being tested is shut, the other is open and the patient is asked to stop breathing).

Don't forget the patient may have a glass eye. Suspect this if visual acuity is zero in one eye and no pupillary reaction is apparent. Lengthy attempts to examine the fundus of a glass eye are embarrassing (and not uncommon).

## *Horner's Syndrome*

If you find a partial ptosis and a constricted pupil (which reacts normally to light), Horner's syndrome is likely (Table 8-42). Proceed as follows.

Look for enophthalmos. Test for a difference in sweating over each eyebrow with the back of your finger (even though your brow is usually more sweaty than the patient's); this only occurs when the lesion is below the carotid bifurcation. Absence of enophthalmos and sweating differences does not exclude the diagnosis of Horner's syndrome.

Examine the appropriate cranial nerves next to exclude the lateral medullary syndrome:

1. Nystagmus (to the side of the lesion).
2. Ipsilateral V (pain and temperature), IX and X cranial nerve lesions.

**Figure 30.** *Eyes*

Sitting up

GENERAL INSPECTION
  Diagnostic facies (Table 8-29)

EYELIDS
  Xanthelasma

CORNEA
  Corneal arcus
  Band keratopathy
  Kayser-Fleischer rings

SCLERA
  Jaundice
  Pallor
  Injection

PTOSIS

EXOPHTHALMOS

LID LAG

NEUROLOGICAL EXAMINATION
  Acuity
    Eye chart—each eye separately
  Fields
    Red pin confrontation—each eye
    Central vision
  Fundi
    Cornea
    Lens
    Humor
    Colour of disc and state of cup
    Retina—vessels, exudates,
      haemorrhages, pigmentation, etc.
  Pupils
    Shape, size
    Light reflex—direct and consensual
    Marcus Gunn phenomenon
    Accommodation
  Eye movements
    III, IV, VI nerves—movement, diplopia,
      nystagmus
    Gaze palsies (e.g., supranuclear
      lesions)
    Fatiguability (myasthenia)
  Corneal reflex (V)

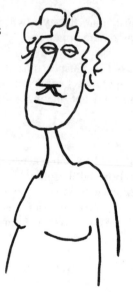

ORBITS
  Palpate—Tenderness
       —Brow (for loss of
         sweating in Horner's
         syndrome)

OTHER
  Depends on findings
    e.g., other cranial nerves,
    long tract signs, urine analysis
    (diabetes)

**Table 8-42.** *Causes of Horner's Syndrome*

1. Carcinoma of the lung apex (usually squamous cell carcinoma)
2. Neck, e.g., thyroid malignancy, trauma
3. Carotid arterial lesion, e.g., carotid aneurysm or dissection, pericarotid tumor
4. Brain stem lesions, e.g., vascular disease (especially the lateral medullary syndrome), syringobulbia, tumour
5. Syringomyelia (rare)

3. Ipsilateral cerebellar signs.
4. CONTRALATERAL pain and temperature loss over the trunk and limbs.

Ask the patient to speak and note any hoarseness (which may be due to recurrent laryngeal nerve palsy from a chest lesion or a cranial nerve lesion).

Look at the hands for clubbing. Test finger abduction to screen for a lower trunk brachial plexus (C8, T1) lesion.

If there are signs of hoarseness or a lower trunk brachial plexus lesion, proceed to a respiratory examination, concentrating on the apices for signs of lung carcinoma (p. 51).

Examine the neck for lymphadenopathy, thyroid carcinoma and a carotid aneurysm or bruit (e.g., fibromuscular dysplasia causing dissection).

As syringomyelia may rarely cause this syndrome, finish off the assessment by examining for dissociated sensory loss. Remember this lesion may cause a BILATERAL Horner's syndrome (a trap for the unwary).

# Notes on The Cranial Nerves

## First (Olfactory) Nerve (p. 205)

*Causes of Anosmia*

Bilateral:

1. Upper respiratory tract infection (commonest).
2. Meningioma of the olfactory groove (late).
3. Ethmoid tumours.
4. Head trauma (including cribriform plate fracture).
5. Meningitis.
6. Hydrocephalus.
7. Congenital, e.g., Kallmann's syndrome (hypogonadotrophic hypogonadism).

Unilateral:

1. Meningioma of the olfactory groove (early).
2. Head trauma.

## Second (Optic) Nerve (p. 206)

*Light Reflex*

Constriction of the pupil in response to light is relayed via the optic nerve and tract, the superior quadrigeminal brachium, the Edinger-Westphal nucleus and its efferent parasympathetic fibres which terminate in the ciliary ganglion. There is no cortical involvement.

*Accommodation Reflex*

Constriction of the pupil with accommodation originates in the cortex (in association with convergence) and is relayed via parasympathetic fibres in the III nerve.

Causes of absent light reflex but intact accommodation reflex:

1. Mid-brain lesion, e.g., Argyll Robertson pupil.
2. Ciliary ganglion lesion (e.g., Adie's pupil).
3. Parinaud's syndrome (p. 217).

Causes of absent convergence but intact light reflex:

Cortical lesion, e.g., cortical blindness, mid-brain lesions (rare).

*Visual Field Defects* (Figure 31)

*Pupil Abnormalities*

Causes of constriction:

1. Horner's syndrome.
2. Argyll Robertson pupil.
3. Pontine lesion (often bilateral but reactive to light).
4. Narcotics.
5. Pilocarpine drops.
6. Old age.

Causes of dilatation:

1. Mydriatics, atropine poisoning or cocaine.
2. Third nerve lesion.
3. Adie's pupil.
4. Iridectomy, lens implant, iritis.
5. Post-trauma, deep coma, cerebral death.
6. Congenital.

## Holmes-Adie Syndrome

Cause:
Lesion in the efferent parasympathetic pathway.

Signs:

1. Dilated pupil.
2. Decreased or absent reaction to light (direct and consensual).
3. Slow or incomplete reaction to accommodation with slow dilatation afterwards.
4. Decreased tendon reflexes.
5. The patients are commonly young women.
6. Denervation super-sensitivity to a weak (e.g., 0.125%) pilocarpine solution.

1.  TUNNEL VISION: concentric diminution
    e.g., glaucoma, papilloedema, syphilis

2.  ENLARGED BLIND SPOT: optic nerve head enlargement

3.  CENTRAL SCOTOMATA: optic nerve head to chiasmal lesion
    e.g., demyelineation, toxic, vascular, nutritional

4.  UNILATERAL FIELD LOSS: optic nerve lesion
    e.g., vascular, tumour

5.  BITEMPORAL HEMIANOPIA: optic chiasm lesion
    e.g., pituitary tumour, sella meningioma

6.  HOMONYMOUS HEMIANOPIA: optic tract to occipital cortex,
    lesion at any point e.g., vascular, tumour
    N.B. incomplete lesion results in macular (central) vision sparing

7.  UPPER QUADRANT HOMONYMOUS HEMIANOPIA: temporal
    lobe lesion e.g., vascular, tumour

8.  LOWER QUADRANT HOMONYMOUS HEMIANOPIA: parietal
    lobe lesion

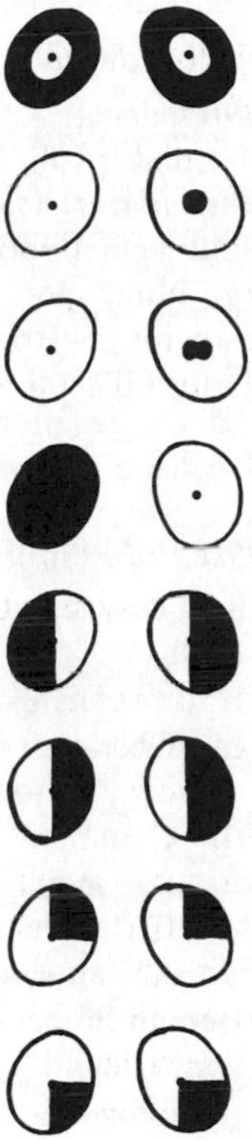

**Figure 31.**   *Visual field defects associated with lesions of the visual system.*

Reproduced and modified, with permission, from Bickerstaff ER Neurological Examination in Clinical Practice.
5th ed. Oxford: Blackwells, 1989

## *Argyll Robertson Pupil*

Cause: Lesion of the iridodilator fibres in the midbrain, as in

1.  Syphilis.
2.  Diabetes mellitus.
3.  Alcoholic neuropathy (rarely).
4.  Other midbrain lesions.

Signs:

1.  Small, irregular, unequal pupil.
2.  No reaction to light.
3.  Prompt reaction to accommodation.
4.  If tabes associated, decreased reflexes.
5.  Mydriatics dilate slowly.

## Papilloedema vs Papillitis

| Papilloedema | Papillitis |
|---|---|
| Optic disc swollen without venous pulsation | Optic disc swollen* |
| Acuity normal (early) | Acuity poor |
| Colour vision normal | Colour vision affected |
| Large blind spot | (particularly red desaturation) |
| Peripheral constriction of visual fields | Large central scotoma |
| Usually bilateral | Pain on eye movement |
| | Onset usually sudden and unilateral |

### Causes of Papilloedema

1. Space-occupying lesion (causing raised intracranial pressure) or a retro-orbital mass.
2. Hydrocephalus (associated with large ventricles).
   (a) Obstructive (block in the ventricle, aqueduct or outlet to fourth ventricle), e.g., tumour.
   (b) Communicating:
       (i) increased formation, e.g., choroid plexus papilloma;
       (ii) decreased absorption, e.g., tumour causing venous compression, sub-arachnoid space obstruction from meningitis.
3. Benign intracranial hypertension (pseudotumour cerebri, associated with small ventricles):
   (a) idiopathic;
   (b) the contraceptive pill;
   (c) Addison's disease;
   (d) drugs, e.g., nitrofurantoin, tetracycline, vitamin A, steroids;
   (e) lateral sinus thrombosis;
   (f) head trauma.
4. Hypertension (grade IV).
5. Central retinal vein thrombosis.
6. Cerebral venous sinus thrombosis.
7. High cerebrospinal fluid protein, e.g., Guillain-Barré syndrome (p. 126).

### Causes of Optic Atrophy

1. Chronic papilloedema or optic neuritis
2. Optic nerve pressure or division
3. Glaucoma
4. Ischaemia
5. Familial, e.g., retinitis pigmentosa, Leber's disease, Friedreich's ataxia.

### Causes of Optic Neuritis

1. Multiple sclerosis (p. 122).
2. Toxic, e.g., ethambutol, chloroquine, nicotine, alcohol.

---

* In retrobulbar neuritis the optic disk becomes pale.

3. Metabolic, e.g., vitamin $B_{12}$ deficiency.
4. Ischaemia, e.g., diabetes mellitus, temporal arteritis, atheroma.
5. Familial, e.g., Leber's disease.
6. Infective, e.g., infectious mononucleosis.

*Causes of Cataract*

1. Old age (senile cataract).
2. Endocrine, e.g., diabetes mellitus, steroids.
3. Hereditary or congenital, e.g., dystrophia myotonica, Refsum's disease.
4. Ocular disease, e.g., glaucoma.
5. Irradiation.
6. Trauma.

*Causes of Ptosis*

With normal pupils:

1. Myasthenia gravis. (p. 124)
2. Myotonic dystrophy.
3. Fascioscapulohumeral dystrophy.
4. Ocular myopathy.
5. Thyrotoxic myopathy.
6. Senile ptosis.
7. Botulism, snake bite.
8. Congenital.

With constricted pupils:

1. Horner's syndrome
2. Tabes dorsalis.

With dilated pupils:

1. III nerve lesion

## Third (Oculomotor) Nerve (p. 206)

*Clinical Features of a Third nerve Palsy*

1. Complete ptosis (partial ptosis may occur with an incomplete lesion).
2. Divergent strabismus (eye 'down and out').
3. Dilated pupil unreactive to direct light (consensual intact) and unreactive to accommodation.

N.B. Always exclude a fourth (trochlear) nerve lesion when a third nerve lesion is present. Do this by tilting the head to the same side as the lesion. The affected eye will intort if the fourth nerve is intact. Or ask the patient to look down and across to the opposite side from the lesion and look for intortion—remember 'SIN': superior (oblique muscle) intorts the eye.

*Aetiology*

Central:

1. Vascular, e.g., brainstem infarction.
2. Tumour.

3. Demyelination (rare).
4. Idiopathic.

N.B. Evidence may include an associated contralateral hemiplegia or occasionally a red nucleus tremor (a coarse, contralateral, slow, proximal limb flap).

Peripheral:

1. Compressive lesions.
    (a) Aneurysm (usually on the posterior communicating artery).
    (b) Tumour causing raised intracranial pressure (dilated pupil occurs early).
    (c) Nasopharyngeal carcinoma.
    (d) Orbital lesions, e.g., Tolosa-Hunt syndrome (superior orbital fissure syndrome—painful lesion of the III, IV, VI and the first division of V cranial nerves).
    (e) Basal meningitis.
2. Infarction, e.g., diabetes mellitus, arteritis (pupil is usually spared).

## Sixth (Abducens) Nerve (p. 206)
### Clinical Features of a Sixth Nerve Palsy
1. Failure of lateral movement.
2. Convergent strabismus.
3. Diplopia—maximal on looking to the affected side. The images are horizontal and parallel to each other. The outermost image is from the affected eye and disappears on covering this eye (this image is also usually more blurred).

### Aetiology
Bilateral:

1. Trauma (head injury).
2. Wernicke's encephalopathy.
3. Raised intracranial pressure.
4. Mononeuritis multiplex.

Unilateral:

1. Central:
    (a) vascular;
    (b) tumour;
    (c) Wernicke's encephalopathy;
    (d) multiple sclerosis (rare).
2. Peripheral:
    (a) trauma;
    (b) idiopathic;
    (c) raised intracranial pressure.

## Eye Movements
With the eye abducted: the elevator is the superior rectus (III nerve). The depressor is the inferior rectus (III nerve).

With the eye adducted: the elevator is the inferior oblique (III nerve). The depressor is the superior oblique (IV nerve).

## Causes of Nystagmus
*Jerky*
1. Horizontal:
    (a) Vestibular lesion [N.B. Chonic lesions cause nystagmus to the side of the lesion (fast component)].
    (b) Cerebellar lesion. (N.B. Unilateral disease causes nystagmus to the side of the lesion).
    (c) Internuclear ophthalmoplegia [N.B. Nystagmus is in the abducting eye, with failure of adduction on the affected side. This is due to a medial longitudinal fasciculus lesion. The commonest cause in young adults with bilateral involvement is multiple sclerosis (p. 123); in the elderly, consider brainstem infarction.]
2. Vertical:
    (a) Brainstem lesion:
        (i)  upgaze nystagmus suggests a lesion in the floor of the IVth ventricle;
        (ii) downgaze nystagmus suggests a foramen magnum lesion.
    (b) Toxic, e.g., phenytoin, alcohol (may also cause horizontal nystagmus)

*Pendular*
1. Retinal (decreased macular vision), e.g., albinism.
2. Congenital.

## Supranuclear Palsy
Loss of vertical upward gaze and sometimes downward gaze. Clinical features (distinguishing from III, IV and VI nerve palsy):

1. Both eyes affected.
2. Pupils fixed, but often unequal.
3. No diplopia.
4. Reflex eye movements (e.g., on flexing and extending the neck) intact.

*Steele-Richardson-Olszewski Syndrome* (progressive supranuclear palsy):

1. Loss of vertical downward gaze first, later vertical upward gaze and finally horizontal gaze.
2. Associated with pseudobulbar palsy, long tract signs, extrapyramidal signs, dementia and neck rigidity.

*Parinaud's Syndrome*

Loss of vertical upward gaze often associated with convergence-retraction nystagmus on attempted convergence and pseudo Argyll-Robertson pupils.

Causes of Parinaud's Syndrome:

1. Pinealoma.
2. Multiple sclerosis (p. 122).
3. Vascular lesions.

## Fifth (Trigeminal) Nerve Palsy (p. 207) (Figure 32)

*Aetiology*

Central (pons, medulla and upper cervical cord):
1. Vascular.
2. Tumour.
3. Syringobulbia.
4. Multiple sclerosis.

Peripheral (posterior fossa):

1. Aneurysm.
2. Tumour (skull base).
3. Chronic meningitis.

Trigeminal ganglion (petrous temporal bone):

1. Acoustic neuroma.
2. Meningioma.
3. Fracture of the middle fossa.

Cavernous sinus (associated III, IV and VI palsies):

1. Aneurysm.
2. Thrombosis.
3. Tumour.

   Other, e.g., Sjögren's syndrome, systemic lupus erythematosus (p. 97).

Remember, if there is:

1. Loss of all sensation in all 3 divisions—consider a lesion at the ganglion or sensory root.
2. Total sensory loss in *1* division—consider a postganglion lesion.
3. Loss of pain but preservation of touch—consider a brainstem or upper cervical cord lesion.
4. Loss of touch but pain sensation is preserved—consider a pontine nuclei lesion.

## Seventh (Facial) Nerve Palsy (p. 207)

*Aetiology*

Upper motor neurone lesion (supranuclear):
1. Vascular.
2. Tumour.

   N.B. Frontal lobe lesions cause weakness of the emotional movements of the face only.

Lower motor neurone lesions

Pontine (often associated with V, VI):

1. Vascular.
2. Tumour.

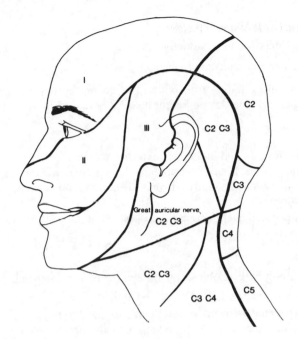

**Figure 32.**  *Dermatomes of the head and neck.*

3. Syringobulbia.
4. Multiple sclerosis.

Posterior fossa:

1. Acoustic neuroma.
2. Meningioma.

Petrous temporal bone:

1. Bell's palsy.
2. Ramsay Hunt syndrome.
3. Otitis media.
4. Fracture.

Parotid:

1. Tumour.
2. Sarcoid.

Causes of bilateral lower motor neurone facial weakness:

1. Guillain-Barré syndrome (p. 126).
2. Bilateral parotid disease (e.g., sarcoid).
3. Mononeuritis multiplex (rare).

   N.B. Myopathy can also cause bilateral facial weakness.

## Eighth (Acoustic) Nerve (p. 208)

To differentiate nerve from conductive deafness:

### Rinne's Test

A 256 Hertz vibrating tuning fork is first placed on the mastoid process, behind the ear, and when the sound is no longer heard it is placed in line with the external meatus.

Results:
1. Normal—the note is audible at the external meatus.
2. Nerve deafness—the note is audible at the external meatus as air and bone conduction are reduced equally, so that air conduction is better (as is normal). Positive result.
3. Conduction (middle ear) deafness—no note is audible at the external meatus. Negative result.

### Weber's Test

A 256 Hertz tuning fork is placed on the centre of the forehead.

Results:
1. Normal—the sound is heard in the centre of the forehead.
2. Nerve deafness—the sound is transmitted to the normal ear.
3. Conduction deafness—the sound is heard to be louder in the abnormal ear.

### Causes of deafness

Nerve (sensorineural) deafness:
1. Tumour, e.g., acoustic neuroma.
2. Trauma, e.g., fracture of the petrous temporal bone, high noise exposure.
3. Toxic, e.g., aspirin, alcohol, streptomycin.
4. Infection, e.g., congenital rubella syndrome, congenital syphilis.
5. Degeneration, e.g., presbyacusis.
6. Brainstem lesions.
7. Vascular disease of the internal auditory artery.

Conduction deafness:

1. Wax.
2. Otitis media.
3. Otosclerosis.
4. Paget's disease of bone (p. 105).

## Ninth (Glossopharyngeal) and Tenth (Vagus) Nerve Palsy (p. 208)

### Aetiology

Central:

1. Vascular, e.g., lateral medullary infarction, due to vertebral or posterior inferior cerebellar artery disease.
2. Tumour.

3. Syringobulbia.
4. Motor neurone disease.

Peripheral—posterior fossa:

1. Aneurysm.
2. Tumour.
3. Chronic meningitis.
4. Guillain-Barré syndrome.

## Twelfth (Hypoglossal) Nerve Palsy (p. 208)

*Aetiology*

Upper Motor Neurone Lesions

1. Vascular.
2. Motor neurone disease.
3. Tumour.
4. Multiple sclerosis (p. 122).

N.B. The syndrome of bilateral upper motor neurone lesions of IX, X and XII is called pseudobulbar palsy.

Lower Motor Neurone Lesions

Unilateral*

Central:

1. Vascular—thrombosis of the vertebral artery.
2. Motor neurone disease.
3. Syringobulbia.

Peripheral (Posterior Fossa):

1. Aneurysm
2. Tumour.
3. Chronic meningitis.
4. Trauma.
5. Arnold Chiari malformation.

N.B. Arnold Chiari malformation is basilar impression of the skull causing lower cranial nerve palsies, cerebellar limb signs (due to tonsillar compression) and upper motor neurone signs in the legs.

Bilateral:

1. Motor neurone disease.
2. Arnold Chiari malformation.
3. Guillain-Barré syndrome.
4. Polio.

---

* It is difficult to detect unilateral lesions as the tongue muscles (except genioglossus) are bilaterally innervated.

### Causes of Multiple Cranial Nerve Palsies

1. Nasopharyngeal carcinoma.
2. Chronic meningitis, e.g., carcinoma, tuberculosis, sarcoidosis.
3. Guillain-Barré syndrome (usually spares I, II and VIII).
4. Brainstem lesion. This is usually due to vascular disease causing crossed sensory or motor paralysis (i.e., cranial nerve signs on one side and contralateral long tract signs). Patients with brainstem glioma may have similar signs and may live for many years.
5. Arnold Chiari malformation.
6. Trauma.
7. Paget's disease.
8. Mononeuritis multiplex, rarely (e.g., diabetes mellitus, p. 235).

## Higher Centres

Examine this patient's higher centres.

### Method (Figure 33)

In this assessment especially, you must be guided by your findings. The introduction is important. For example, if you are told the patient also presents with right-sided weakness, you should concentrate on looking for dominant parietal lobe signs.

Shake the patient's hand, noting any obvious focal weakness, and introduce yourself. Tell him you will be asking him some questions.

First, ask if the patient is right or left handed. Then ask questions about orientation (person, place and time). Ask name, the present location and the date.

This also allows you to test for speech abnormality. Receptive dysphasia should be obvious, as should severe expressive dysphasia. Assess any nominal dysphasia by asking the patient to name some objects, e.g., your watch, a pen (Table 8-43).

Assess the parietal lobes next. Begin with the dominant parietal lobe as Gerstmann's syndrome is common in examinations. Examine for *acalculia* (test mental arithmetic), *agraphia* (inability to write), *left-right disorientation* (e.g., by asking the patient to put right palm on left ear, then vice versa), and *finger agnosia* (inability to name individual fingers). This is due to a left angular gyrus lesion in right-handed and about half of left-handed patients. (A mnemonic for Gerstmann's syndrome is 'ALF').

Test general parietal functions (involving either lobe). Examine for sensory and visual inattention. Also test for agraphism (inability to appreciate numbers drawn on the palm) and asterognosis (inability to name objects placed in the hand). Test for sensory apraxia if appropriate. Assess constructional apraxia by asking the patient to draw a clock face and fill in the numbers.

The major specific non-dominant parietal dysfunction is dressing apraxia. This can be tested by putting the patient's pyjama top inside out and asking him to put it on correctly.

Assess memory, both short and long term. This is a medial temporal lobe

**Figure 33.** *Higher Centres*

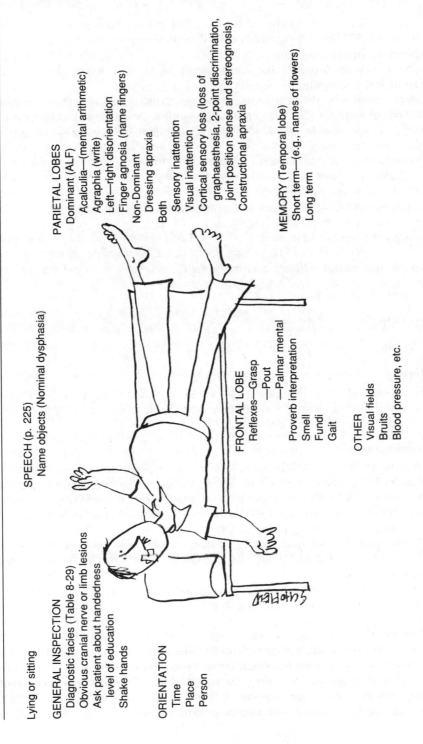

Lying or sitting

GENERAL INSPECTION
Diagnostic facies (Table 8-29)
Obvious cranial nerve or limb lesions
Ask patient about handedness
    level of education
Shake hands

ORIENTATION
Time
Place
Person

SPEECH (p. 225)
Name objects (Nominal dysphasia)

PARIETAL LOBES
Dominant (ALF)
    Acalculia—(mental arithmetic)
    Agraphia (write)
    Left—right disorientation
    Finger agnosia (name fingers)
Non-Dominant
    Dressing apraxia
Both
    Sensory inattention
    Visual inattention
    Cortical sensory loss (loss of
        graphaesthesia, 2-point discrimination,
        joint position sense and stereognosis)
    Constructional apraxia

MEMORY (Temporal lobe)
Short term—(e.g., names of flowers)
Long term

FRONTAL LOBE
Reflexes—Grasp
        —Pout
        —Palmar mental
Proverb interpretation
Smell
Fundi
Gait

OTHER
Visual fields
Bruits
Blood pressure, etc.

function. Ask the patient to remember the name of three flowers (e.g., rose, orchid and tulip—ROT for those candidates with a poor memory) and repeat them immediately. Then assess long-term memory, e.g., by asking when World War II finished. Ask the names of the flowers again at the end of your higher centres examination.

Test frontal lobe problems, first by assessing the primitive reflexes, normally not present in adults. The grasp reflex, pout reflex, and palmar-mental reflex are usually all that need be tested. Then ask for interpretation of a common proverb, e.g., 'a rolling stone gathers no moss'. Test for anosmia (cranial nerve I) and gait apraxia (a frontal gait abnormality is marked by gross unsteadiness in walking—the feet typically behave as if glued to the floor resulting in a wide-based shuffling gait). Look at the fundi to exclude the rare Foster Kennedy syndrome (optic atrophy on the side of the lesion and papilloedema in the opposite fundus) if there is evidence of a frontal lobe lesion.

Any abnormality of the parietal, temporal or occipital lobes may cause a characteristic visual field loss. This should be tested if appropriate, at the conclusion of your examination. Other important signs to look for are carotid bruits, hypertension and relevant focal neurological signs.

# Speech

Assess this patient's speech.

## Method

Immediately ask the patient to state his name, age and present location. Then ask him to say 'British Constitution'. By now you should have decided if the problem is dysphasia, dysarthria or dysphonia.

## Dysphasia

If the speech is fluent, but conveys information imperfectly often with paraphrasic errors (e.g., 'treen for train'), the main possibilities are nominal, receptive and conductive aphasia. Test for these by asking the patient to name objects, repeat a statement after you and then follow commands. Then ask him to read and write if the above are abnormal (Table 8-43).

If the speech is slow and non-fluent (hesitant), exactly the same procedure is followed, but an expressive aphasia is likely. At the end ask to assess for a hemiparesis (Table 8-43).

Remember large lesions may cause global aphasia, with inability to comprehend or speak, plus hemiparesis (Table 8-44).

## Dysarthria

This is a disorder of articulation with no disorder of the content of speech. Consider cerebellar disease and lower cranial nerve lesions particularly. Cerebellar speech is slurred or 'scanning' (i.e. irregular and staccato). Pseudobulbar palsy causes slow, hesitant, hollow-sounding speech with a harsh, strained voice, whilst bulbar palsy causes nasal speech with imprecise articulation.

**Table 8-43.** *Examination of Dysphasia*

**Fluent Speech (Receptive, Conductive or Nominal Dysphasia usually)**
1. Naming of objects. Patients with nominal, conductive or receptive aphasia all name objects poorly
2. Repetition. Conductive and receptive aphasics cannot repeat.
3. Comprehension. Only receptive aphasic patients cannot follow commands (verbal or written).
4. Reading. Conductive and receptive aphasic patients have difficulty.
5. Writing. Conductive aphasic patients have impaired writing (dysgraphia) while receptive aphasic patients have abnormal content. Dysgraphia may also occur with dominant frontal lobe lesions.

**Non-fluent Speech (usually Expressive Aphasia)\***
1. Naming of objects. Poor (but may be better than spontaneous speech).
2. Repetition. May be possible with great effort. Phrase repetition (e.g., 'no ifs, ands or buts') is poor.
3. Comprehension. Normal (written and verbal commands are followed).
4. Writing. Dysgraphia may be present.
5. Look for hemiparesis. Arm more affected than leg.

\* N.B. As the patient is aware of his deficit he is often frustrated and depressed.


**Table 8-44.** *The Sites of Lesions in Aphasia*

*Receptive Aphasia:*
Wernicke's area—posterior part of first temporal gyrus in the dominant lobe.

*Expressive Aphasia*
Broca's area—posterior part of the third frontal gyrus.

*Conductive Aphasia:*
Arcuate fasciculus and/or conducting fibres (temporal lobe).

*Nominal Aphasia:*
Angular gyrus (temporal lobe)—small localized lesion. Other causes: encephalopathies (metabolic, toxic), pressure effects from a distant space-occupying lesion, recovery phase from any dysphasia.


Ask the patient to say 'British Constitution', 'West Register Street', 'Me Me Me' and 'Lah Lah Lah'. If the speech is cerebellar, go on to this system (p. 245). If palsy of a lower cranial nerve is likely, examine the cranial nerves carefully. Don't forget to elicit the jaw jerk. Look in the mouth too for ulceration or other local lesions.

Less common causes of dysarthria include extrapyramidal disease (p. 249) and myopathies (p. 243).

## *Dysphonia*

This is huskiness of the voice from a laryngeal disorder, recurrent laryngeal nerve palsy or focal dystonia. Assess the quality of the cough too.

## Upper Limbs

This patient has noticed weakness in the arms. Please examine.

### Method (Figure 34)

Look at the whole patient briefly. Note particularly evidence of a myopathic face, Parkinsonian features or stroke.

Shake the patient's hand firmly and introduce yourself. If he cannot let go, you have made the diagnosis (myotonia, usually due to dystrophia myotonica). Ask the patient to sit over the side of the bed facing you.

Examine the MOTOR SYSTEM systematically every time.

Inspect first for wasting (both proximally and distally) and fasciculations. Don't forget to include the shoulder girdle in your inspection (p. 229).

Ask the patient to hold both hands out with the arms extended and close his eyes. Look for drifting of one or both arms. There are only 3 causes for this drift:

1. Upper motor neurone weakness (usually downwards due to muscle weakness)
2. Cerebellar lesion (usually upwards due to hypotonia)
3. Posterior column loss (any direction due to joint position sense loss).

Also note any tremor and pseudoathetosis due to proprioceptive loss.

Feel the muscle bulk next, both proximally and distally, and note any muscle tenderness. Tap the muscles with your tendon hammer or finger to elicit fasciculation. In the presence of wasting and weakness, fasciculation indicates lower motor neurone degeneration.

Test tone at the wrists and elbows by moving the joints, at varying velocities. Assess power next.

### Shoulder

Abduction (C5,6): tell the patient to abduct his arms with the elbows flexed and not to let you push them down.

Adduction (C6–8): tell him to adduct his arms with the elbows flexed and not let you separate them.

### Elbow

Flexion (C5,6): tell him to bend his elbow and pull, so as not to let you straighten it.

Extension (C7,8): tell him to bend his elbow and push, so as not to let you bend it.

### Wrist

Flexion (C6,7): tell him to bend his wrist and not let you straighten it.

Extension (C7,8): tell him to straighten his wrist and not to let you bend it.

### Finger

Extension (C7,C8): tell him to straighten his fingers and to not let you push them down.

Flexion (C7,8): tell him to squeeze two of your fingers.

**Figure 34.** *Upper Limbs Neurologically*

GENERAL INSPECTION
Diagnostic facies (Table 8-29)
Scars
Skin, e.g., neurofibromata, cafe-au-lait
Abnormal movements

SENSORY SYSTEM
Pain (pin prick)
Vibration (128 Hz tuning fork)
Proprioception—DIP joint (each hand)
Light touch (cotton wool)

SHAKE HANDS

MOTOR SYSTEM
Inspect arms, shoulder girdle—extend both
arms:
    Wasting
    Fasciculation
    Tremor
    Drift
Palpate
    Muscle bulk
    Muscle tenderness
    Tap—for fasciculation
Tone
    Wrist
    Elbow
Power
    Shoulder
    Elbow
    Wrist
    Fingers
    Ulnar, median nerve function
Reflexes
    Biceps
    Triceps
    Supinator
    Finger
Coordination
    Finger-nose test—intention tremor,
        past pointing
    Dysdiadochokinesis
    Rebound

OTHER
Thickened nerves (wrist, elbow)
Axillae
Neck
Lower limbs
Cranial nerves
Urine analysis, etc.

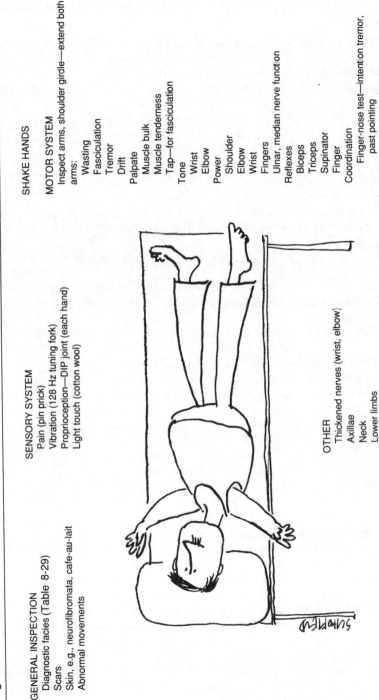

DIP = distal interphalangeal joint

Abduction (C8,T1): tell him to spread out his fingers and not let you push them together.

You should not be able to overcome a normal patient's power. Grade the power.

Next test for an ulnar lesion (loss of finger abduction and adduction) and a median nerve lesion (loss of thumb abduction) (p. 237).

Examine the reflexes:

Biceps (C5,6)—biceps muscle.
Triceps (C7,8)—triceps muscle
Supinator (C5,6)—brachioradialis muscle.
*Inverted supinator jerk* (associated with an absent biceps and exaggerated triceps jerk, indicating an intraspinal lesion compressing the spinal cord and nerve roots at C5,6)
Finger (C8).

Assess coordination with finger/nose testing and look for dysdiadochokinesis and rebound (p. 245).

Motor weakness can be due to an upper motor neurone lesion, lower motor neurone lesion or myopathy.

If there is evidence of a lower motor neurone lesion, consider anterior horn cell, nerve root and brachial plexus lesions, peripheral nerve lesions, or a motor peripheral neuropathy.

Examine the SENSORY SYSTEM after motor testing, because this can be time-consuming.

First test the spinothalamic pathway (pain and temperature).

Use a new blunt pin. One candidate accidentally pricked his own finger during the examination with a sharp pin. By the time he stopped bleeding his short case time was up. In case you believe this might be a good ploy, the candidate failed.

First demonstrate to the patient the sharpness of the pin on the anterior chest wall or forehead. Then ask him to close his eyes and tell you if the sensation is sharp or dull. Start proximally and test each dermatome. As you are assessing, try to fit any sensory loss into dermatomal (cord or nerve root lesion) (Figure 35), peripheral nerve, peripheral neuropathy (glove) or hemisensory (cortical or cord) distribution. Also remember that 'cape' sensory loss suggests syringomyelia while 'shield' sensory loss may occur with syphilis. It is not usually necessary to test temperature perception in the examination.

Next test the posterior column pathway (vibration and proprioception).

Use a 128 Hertz tuning fork to assess vibration sense. Place this when vibrating on the ulnar head at the wrist when the patient has his eyes closed and ask if he can feel it. If so, ask him to tell you when the vibration ceases and then stop the vibrations. If the patient has deficient sensation, test at the elbow, then shoulder.

Examine proprioception first with the distal interphalangeal joint of the index finger. When the patient has his eye open grasp his distal phalanx from the sides and move it up and down to demonstrate, then ask him to close his eyes and repeat the manoeuvres. Normally, movement through even a few degrees is detectable, and he can tell if it is up or down. If there is an abnormality, proceed to test the wrist and elbows similarly.

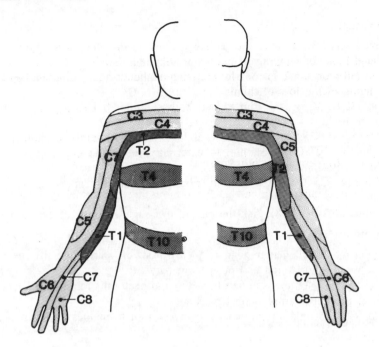

**Figure 35.** *Dermatomes of the upper limb and trunk.*

Reproduced and modified with permission, from Lance JW, McLeod JG A Physiological Approach to Clinical Neurology. 3rd ed. London: Butterworths, 1981

Test light touch with cotton wool. Touch the skin lightly (do not stroke) in each dermatome.

Feel for thickened nerves—ulnar at the elbow, median at the wrist, and radial at the wrist—and feel the axillae if there is evidence of a plexus lesion. Don't forget to mention any scars that may be present. Finally examine the neck if relevant.

To confirm a diagnosis, it may be necessary to examine further afield. Ask the examiners if you can do this. For example, if there is evidence of motor neurone disease, assess the lower limbs as well as the tongue. If there is evidence of a C5,6 root lesion, assess the lower limbs neurologically and the neck for cervical spondylosis.

## Shoulder Girdle Examination

Examine this man's shoulder girdle.

### *Methods*

This is likely to be a muscular dystrophy or a root lesion.

Proceed by inspecting each muscle, palpating its bulk and testing function as follows.

From the back:

1. Trapezius (XI,C3,C4): Ask the patient to elevate the shoulders against resistance and look for winging of the upper scapula.
2. Serratus anterior (C5–C7): Ask him to push his hands against the wall and look for winging of the lower scapula.
3. Rhomboids (C4,C5): Ask him to pull both shoulder blades together with his hands on his hips.
4. Supraspinatus: (C5,C6): Ask him to abduct his arms against resistance.
5. Infraspinatus: (C5,C6): Ask him to externally rotate the upper arms against resistance with his arms at his side.
6. Teres major (C5–C7): Ask him to internally rotate the upper arms against resistance.
7. Latissimus dorsi (C7,C8): Ask the patient to cough and palpate on both sides.

From the front:

1. Pectoralis major, clavicular head (C5–C8): Ask the patient to lift the upper arms above the horizontal and push them forward.
2. Pectoralis major, sternocostal part (C6–T1) and pectoralis minor (C7): Ask him to adduct the upper arms against resistance.
3. Deltoid (C5,C6) (and circumflex nerve): Ask him to abduct the arms against resistance.

## Lower Limbs

Examine this patient's lower limbs neurologically.

### *Method* (Figure 36)

Test the gait first (p. 245). Ask the examiners if this is possible—sometimes they will not let you examine the gait.

Note the general appearance. Especially look for upper limb girdle wasting and the presence of a urinary catheter.

Have the patient lie in bed with the legs entirely exposed. Place a towel over the groin.

Look for muscle wasting and fasciculation. Note any tremor. Tap the quadriceps and calves with your patella hammer or finger for fasciculation. Feel the muscle bulk of the quadriceps and run your hand up each shin, feeling for wasting of the anterior tibial muscles.

Test tone at the knees and ankles. Test clonus at this time. Push the patella sharply downwards. Sustained rhythmical contractions indicate an upper motor neurone lesion. Also test the ankle by sharply dorsiflexing the foot with the knee bent and the thigh externally rotated.

Assess power next.

### *Hip*

Flexion (L2,3): ask the patient to lift up his straight leg and not to let you push it down (having placed your hand above his knee).

**Figure 36.** *Lower Limbs Neurologically*

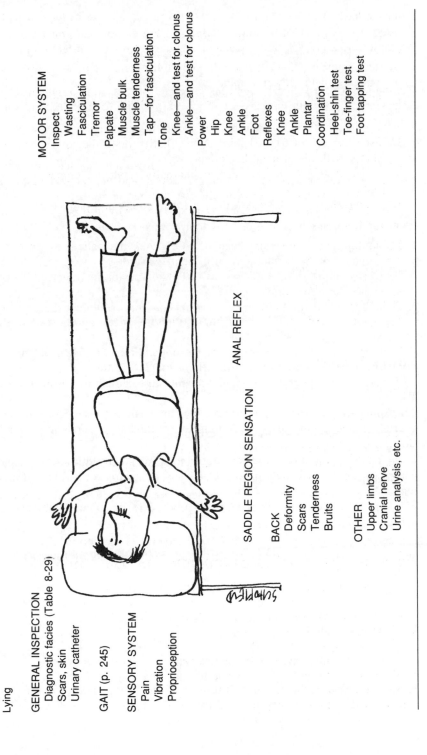

Lying

GENERAL INSPECTION
Diagnostic facies (Table 8-29)
Scars, skin
Urinary catheter

GAIT (p. 245)

SENSORY SYSTEM
Pain
Vibration
Proprioception

SADDLE REGION SENSATION

BACK
Deformity
Scars
Tenderness
Bruits

ANAL REFLEX

OTHER
Upper limbs
Cranial nerve
Urine analysis, etc.

MOTOR SYSTEM
Inspect
    Wasting
    Fasciculation
    Tremor
Palpate
    Muscle bulk
    Muscle tenderness
    Tap—for fasciculation
Tone
    Knee—and test for clonus
    Ankle—and test for clonus
Power
    Hip
    Knee
    Ankle
    Foot
Reflexes
    Knee
    Ankle
    Plantar
Coordination
    Heel-shin test
    Toe-finger test
    Foot tapping test

Extension (L5,S1,2): ask him to keep his leg down and not to let you pull it up.
Abduction (L4,L5,S1): ask him to abduct his leg and not let you push it in.
Adduction (L2,3,4): ask him to keep his leg adducted and not let you push it out.

*Knee*

Flexion (L5,S1): ask him to bend his knee and not let you straighten it.
Extension (L3,4): with the knee slightly bent, ask him to straighten the knee and
    not let you bend it.

*Ankle*

Plantar flexion (S1): ask him to push his foot down and not let you push it up.
Dorsiflexion (L4,5): ask him to bring his foot up and not let you push it down.
Eversion (L5,S1): ask him to evert the foot against resistance; loss of this may
    also indicate a common peroneal (lateral popliteal) nerve palsy (p. 238).
Inversion (L4): ask him to invert his foot against resistance.

Elicit the reflexes:

Knee (L3,4)—quadriceps muscle.
Ankle (L5,S1)—calf muscle.
Plantar response (S1).

Test coordination with the heel/shin test, toe/finger test and tapping of the feet
(p. 248).

Examine the sensory system as for the upper limbs (p. 228): pin prick, then
vibration and proprioception and then light touch (Figure 37).

If there is a peripheral sensory loss attempt to establish a sensory level on the
abdomen.

Examine the saddle region sensation. Test the anal reflex (S4,S5); if intact, there
is brief contraction of the external sphincter of the anus to scratching the perianal
skin.

Go to the back. Look for deformity, scars and neurofibromata. Palpate for
tenderness over the vertebral bodies and auscultate for bruits. Test straight leg
raising.

It may be relevant to ask if you can proceed to the upper limbs and cranial
nerves.

# Notes on Neurological Examination of The Limbs

*Grading Muscle Power*
0. Complete paralysis.
1. Flicker of contraction.
2. Movement with NO gravity.
3. Movement with gravity only (any resistance stops movement).
4. Movement with gravity plus some resistance.
5. Normal power.

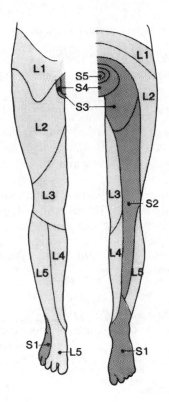

**Figure 37.** *Dermatomes of the lower limb.*

Reproduced, with permission, from Lance JW, McLeod JG A Physiological Approach to Clinical Neurology. 3rd ed. London: Butterworths, 1981

## Signs of a Lower Motor Neurone Lesion

1. Weakness.
2. Wasting.
3. Hypotonicity.
4. Decreased or absent reflexes.
5. Fasciculation (prominent in anterior horn cell diseases usually).

## Signs of an Upper Motor Neurone Lesion

1. Weakness in an 'upper motor neurone pattern'. Upper limb—abductor and extensor muscles weak—e.g., shoulder abduction, elbow and wrist extensors are affected. Lower limb—flexor and adductor muscles weak—e.g., hip flexion, knee flexion, ankle dorsiflexion affected.
2. Spasticity.

3. Clonus.
4. Increased reflexes and extensor plantar response.

## An Approach to Peripheral Neuropathy

This may be sensory (glove and stocking), motor or both.

### Common Causes of Peripheral Neuropathy ('DAM, IT, BICH')

1. Drugs and toxins, e.g., isoniazid, vincristine, phenytoin, nitrofurantoin, cis-platinum, amiodarone, large doses of vitamin $B_6$, heavy metals.
2. Alcohol (with or without vitamin $B_1$ deficiency); amyloid.
3. Metabolic, e.g., diabetes (p. 108), uraemia (p. 113), hypothyroidism (p. 188), porphyria.
4. Infection associated, eg., Guillain-Barré syndrome (p. 126).
5. Tumour, e.g., lung carcinoma (p. 51).
6. $B_{12}$, $B_1$, or $B_6$ deficiency.
7. Idiopathic.
8. Connective tissue diseases or vasculitis, e.g., systemic lupus erythematosus (p. 97), polyarteritis nodosa.
9. Hereditary.

### Causes of a Predominant Motor Neuropathy

1 Guillain-Barré syndrome and chronic inflammatory demyelinating polyradiculo-neuropathy (CIDP).
2. Hereditary motor and sensory neuropathy (Charcot-Marie-Tooth disease) (p. 236).
3. Acute intermittent porphyria.
4. Lead poisoning.
5. Diabetes mellitus.

   N.B. Motor neurone disease and neuromuscular junction disorders must always be considered.

### Causes of a Predominant Sensory Neuropathy (Sensory Neuronopathy)

This is unusual and results in sensory ataxia and pseudoathetosis. Causes include:

1. Carcinoma, e.g., lung, ovary, breast.
2. Paraproteinemia (p. 90).
3. Vitamin $B_6$ intoxication.
4. Sjögren's syndrome.
5. Diabetes mellitus.
6. Syphilis.
7. Vitamin $B_{12}$ deficiency (occasionally).
8. Idiopathic.

### Causes of a Painful Peripheral Neuropathy

1. Diabetes mellitus.
2. Alcohol.
3. Vitamin $B_{12}$ or $B_1$ deficiency.

4. Carcinoma.
5. Porphyria.
6. Arsenic or thallium poisoning.
7. Hereditary (many are not painful).

N.B. Burning soles of the feet can be caused by a painful peripheral neuropathy, tarsal tunnel syndrome, or an S1 lesion.

## Mononeuritis Multiplex

Mononeuritis multiplex refers to separate involvement of more than one peripheral or rarely cranial nerve, e.g., a common peroneal nerve palsy plus an axillary nerve palsy.

Common causes of mononeuritis multiplex:

Acute (usually vascular):

1. Diabetes mellitus.
2. Polyarteritis nodosa or connective tissue diseases, e.g., systemic lupus erythematosus, rheumatoid arthritis (p. 92).

Chronic:

1. Multiple compressive neuropathies, especially with joint deforming arthritis.
2. Sarcoidosis (p. 58).
3. Acromegaly (p. 192).
4. Leprosy.
5. Lyme disease.
6. Carcinoma (rare).
7. Idiopathic.

## Causes of Thickened Nerves:

1. Hypertrophic neuropathy (autosomal dominant or recessive).
2. Acromegaly.
3. Chronic inflammatory polyradiculoneuropathy.
4. Amyloid.
5. Leprosy.
6. Others, e.g., sarcoid, hereditary motor and sensory neuropathy, neurofibromatosis.

## Fasciculation

Fasciculation is *not* always motor neurone disease.
Causes of fasciculation:

1. Motor neurone disease.
2. Motor root compression.
3. Malignant neuropathy.
4. Any motor neuropathy (less commonly).

N.B. Myokymia resembles benign coarse fasciculation of the same muscle group, e.g., eyelids. Electromyographic myokymia can occur in multiple sclerosis, brainstem neoplasm, Bell's palsy, radiculopathy or radiation plexopathy.

### An Important Syndrome

*Hereditary Motor and Sensory Neuropathy—HMSN Type I*
(Charcot-Marie-Tooth disease: autosomal dominant)
Clinical features:

1. Pes cavus (short, high-arched feet with hammer toes).
2. Distal muscle atrophy due to peripheral nerve degeneration. Not usually extending above the elbows or above the middle one-third of the thighs.
3. Absent reflexes.
4. Slight to no sensory loss in the limbs.
5. Thickened nerves.
6. Optic atrophy; Argyll Robertson pupils (rare).

### An Approach to Brachial Plexus Lesions

Complete lesion:

1. Lower motor neurone signs affect the whole arm.
2. Sensory loss (whole limb).
3. Horner's syndrome (an important clue) (p. 209).

N.B. This is often painful. Remember always to feel for axillary lymphadenopathy at the end of your examination.

Upper (Erb Duchenne) (C5,C6) lesion:
1. Loss of shoulder movement and elbow flexion—hand is held in the 'waiter's tip' position.
2. Sensory loss is present over the lateral aspect of the arm and forearm.

Lower (Klumpke) (C8,T1) lesion:

1. True claw hand with paralysis of all the intrinsic muscles.
2. Sensory loss along the ulnar side of the hand and forearm.
3. Horner's syndrome.

Cervical rib syndrome:

1. Weakness and wasting of the small muscles of the hand (true claw hand).
2. C8 and T1 sensory loss.
3. Unequal radial pulses and blood pressures.
4. Subclavian bruit and loss of the pulse on arm manoeuvring (this sign is often also present in normal persons).
5. Palpable cervical rib in the neck (uncommon).

### Important Peripheral Nerves

*Radial Nerve (C5–C8) Lesion*
Clinical features:

1. Wrist and finger drop (wrist flexion normal).
2. Triceps loss (elbow extension loss) if lesion above the elbow.
3. Sensory loss over the anatomical snuff box.

*Median Nerve (C6–T1) Lesion*

This nerve supplies all muscles on the front of the forearm except flexor carpi ulnaris and half of flexor digitorum profundus. It also supplies the following short muscles of the hand (LOAF):

L—Lateral two lumbricals
O—Opponens pollicis
A—Abductor pollicis brevis
F—Flexor pollicis brevis

Clinical features:

1. Loss of abductor pollicis brevis with a lesion at the wrist. Pen touching test: with the hand flat, ask the patient to abduct the thumb vertically to touch the examiner's pen.
2. Loss of flexor digitorum sublimus with a lesion in or above the cubital fossa. Ochsner's clasping test: ask the patient to clasp the hands firmly together—the index finger on the affected side fails to flex.
3. Sensory loss over the thumb, index, middle and lateral half of the ring finger (palmar aspect only).

N.B. Causes of carpal tunnel syndrome:

1. Idiopathic.
2. Arthropathy, e.g., rheumatoid arthritis (p. 92).
3. Endocrine disease, e.g., myxoedema (p. 188), acromegaly (p. 192).
4. Pregnancy; the contraceptive pill.
5. Trauma and overuse.

*Ulnar Nerve (C8–T1) Lesion*

Clinical features:

1. Wasting of the intrinsic muscles of the hand (except LOAF muscles).
2. Weak finger abduction and adduction (loss of interosseous muscles).
3. Ulnar claw-like hand. (N.B. A higher lesion causes less deformity, as an above-the-elbow lesion also causes loss of flexor digitorum profundus.)
4. Froment's sign: ask the patient to grasp a piece of paper between the thumb and lateral aspect of the forefinger with each hand—the affected thumb will flex (loss of thumb adductor).
5. Sensory loss over the little and medial half of ring finger (both palmar and dorsal aspects).

*Wasting of the Small Muscles of the Hand*

Examine as for the upper limbs and make sure you feel the pulses and examine the neck, unless the causes is very obvious, e.g., rheumatoid arthritis.
Causes:

1. Nerve lesions:
   (a) Median and ulnar nerve lesions
   (b) Brachial plexus lesions

    (c) Peripheral motor neuropathy (in the examination, don't forget hereditary motor and sensory neuropathy).
2. Anterior horn cell disease:
    (a) Motor neurone disease
    (b) Polio
    (c) Spinal muscular atrophies (e.g., Kugelberg-Welander disease).
3. Myopathy:
    (a) Dystrophia myotonica—forearms more affected than the hands
    (b) Distal myopathy.
4. Spinal cord lesions:
    (a) Syringomyelia
    (b) Cervical spondylosis with compression of C8 segment
    (c) Other, e.g., tumour.
5. Trophic disorders:
    (a) Arthropathies (disuse)
    (b) Ischaemia, including vasculitis.
    (c) Shoulder-hand syndrome.

N.B. Distinguishing an ulnar nerve lesion from a C8 root/lower trunk brachial plexus lesion—remember the sensory loss of a C8 lesion extends proximal to the wrist, and the thenar muscles are involved with a C8 root or lower trunk brachial plexus lesion. Distinguishing a C8 root from a lower trunk brachial plexus lesion is difficult clinically, but the presence of Horner's syndrome or an axillary mass suggests the brachial plexus is affected.

*Femoral Nerve (L2,3,4) Lesion*
Clinical features:

1. Weakness of knee extension (quadriceps paralysis).
2. Slight hip flexion weakness.
3. Preserved adductor strength.
4. Loss of knee jerk.
5. Sensory loss involving the inner aspect of the thigh and leg.

*Sciatic Nerve (L4,5,S1,2) Lesion*
Clinical features:

1. Weakness of knee flexion (hamstrings involved).
2. Loss of power of all muscles below the knee causing a foot drop, so the patient may be able to walk, but cannot stand on his toes.
3. Knee jerk intact.
4. Loss of ankle jerk and plantar response.
5. Sensory loss along the posterior thigh and total loss below the knee.

*Common Peroneal (Lateral Popliteal) Nerve (L4,5) Lesion*
Clinical features:

1. Foot drop and loss of foot eversion only.

2. Minimal sensory loss (minimal loss over the lateral aspect of the dorsum of the
   foot).
   N.B. The reflexes are normal.

Distinguishing a common peroneal and L5 root lesion—the L5 lesion causes
weakness of knee flexion, loss of foot inversion as well as eversion, with a sensory
loss involving the L5 distribution sparing the little toe and sole.

### Lateral Cutaneous Nerve of the Thigh Lesion

Meralgia paraesthetica is due to compression of this nerve which may cause sensory
loss and/or hyperaesthesia over the lateral aspect of the thigh, but no motor loss.

### Causes of Foot Drop:

1. Common peroneal nerve palsy.
2. Sciatic nerve palsy.
3. Lumbosacral plexus lesion.
4. L4,L5 root lesion.
5. Peripheral motor neuropathy.
6. Distal myopathy.
7. Motor neurone disease.
8. Precentral gyrus lesion.

N.B. Remember, if there is a foot drop, test the ankle jerk carefully. As a very
rough rule of thumb, if it is absent, an S1 lesion should be suspected; if it is
normal, a common peroneal palsy should be considered; if it is increased, an upper
motor neurone lesion is likely.

# Notes on Spinal Cord Lesions

## Assessment of the Paraplegic Patient

1. Sensory level:
   Patterns of sensory loss depend on the level and type of lesion.
   Consider:
   (a) Cord compression causes a loss of all modalities bilaterally below the level
       involved (note: extrinsic compression may spare the perineum), while
       radicular pain and lower motor neurone weakness are present at the level
       of spinal compression.
   (b) Transverse myelitis.
   (c) Anterior spinal artery occlusion (posterior column function is spared).
2. Back examination:
   e.g., deformity, tenderness or bruits may provide clues about the underlying
   disease process.
3. Arm involvement:
   Consider:
   (a) Cervical spondylosis.
   (b) Syringomyelia.
   (c) Motor neurone disease.
   (d) Multiple sclerosis (p. 122).

4. Cranial nerve lesions:
   Consider:
   (a) Motor neurone disease.
   (b) Multiple sclerosis.
5. Peripheral neuropathy:
   Consider:
   (a) Vitamin $B_{12}$ deficiency.
   (b) Friedreich's ataxia.
   (c) Carcinoma.
   (d) Hereditary spastic paraplegia.
   (e) Syphilis.
6. Cerebral lesions.

N.B. Intracranial lesions, e.g., parasagittal meningioma, cause paraplegia in EXTENSION only, whilst spinal cord lesions cause paraplegia in FLEXION or EXTENSION (i.e., flexor reflexes are released with spinal lesions).

## Important Motor and Reflex Changes of Spinal Cord and Conus Compression

Lower motor neurone signs occur at the level of the root lesion and upper motor neurone signs occur below the lesion.

Upper cervical:

Upper motor neurone signs in the upper and lower limbs.

C5:

Lower motor neurone weakness and wasting of the rhomboids, deltoids, biceps and brachioradialis.
Upper motor neurone signs affect the rest of the upper and all the lower limbs.
The biceps jerk is lost.
The supinator jerk is 'inverted' (tapping the biceps tendon causes triceps contraction).

C8:

Lower motor neurone weakness and wasting of the intrinsic muscles of the hand.
Upper motor neurone signs in the lower limbs.

Midthoracic:

Intercostal paralysis.
Loss of upper abdominal reflexes at T7 and T8.
Upper motor neurone signs in the lower limbs.

T10–T11:

Loss of the lower abdominal reflexes and upward displacement of the umbilicus.
Upper motor neurone signs in the lower limbs.

L1:

Cremasteric reflexes lost (normal abdominal reflexes).
Upper motor neurone signs in the lower limbs.

L4:

Lower motor neurone weakness and wasting of the quadriceps. Knee jerks lost.
Ankle jerks may be hyperreflexic with an extensor plantar response (upgoing
   toes), but more often the whole conus is involved, causing a lower motor neurone
   lesion.

L5 and S1:

Lower motor neurone weakness of knee flexion and hip extension (S1) and
   abduction (L5) plus calf and foot muscles.
Knee jerks present.
No ankle jerks or plantar response.
Anal reflex present.

S3–S4:

No anal reflex.
Saddle sensory loss.
Normal lower limbs
N.B. Look for a urinary catheter.

## *Important Syndromes*

*Subacute Combined Degeneration of the Cord (B$_{12}$ Deficiency)*

Clinical features:

1. Symmetrical posterior column loss (vibration and position sense) causing an
   ataxic gait.
2. Symmetrical upper motor neurone signs in the lower limbs with absent ankle
   reflexes. Knee reflexes may be absent or, more often, exaggerated.
3. Peripheral sensory neuropathy (less common and mild).
4. Optic atrophy.
5. Dementia.

   The combination of upper motor neurone signs causing an extensor plantar response plus peripheral neuropathy causing loss of knee and ankle jerks is a dis-
tinctive pattern.

   Causes of an extensor plantar response plus absent ankle jerks include:

1. Subacute combined degeneration of the cord (B$_{12}$ deficiency).
2. Conus medullaris lesion.
3. Combination of an upper motor neurone lesion with cauda equina compression
   or peripheral neuropathy.
4. Syphilis (tabo-paresis).
5. Friedreich's ataxia.
6. Diabetes mellitus (uncommon) (p. 108).
7. Adrenoleukodystrophy or metochromatic leukodystrophy (p. 197).
8. Motor neurone disease (rare).

*Brown-Séquard Syndrome*
Clinical features:

  Motor changes:

1. Upper motor neurone signs below the hemisection on the SAME side as the lesion.
2. Lower motor neurone signs at the level of the hemisection on the SAME side.

Sensory changes:

1. Pain and temperature loss on the OPPOSITE side of the lesion.
   N.B. The upper level of sensory loss is usually a few segments below the level of the lesion.
2. Vibration and proprioception loss occurs on the SAME side.
3. Light touch is often normal.

Common causes:

1. Multiple sclerosis (p. 122).
2. Angioma.
3. Glioma.
4. Trauma.
5. Myelitis.
6. Postradiation myelopathy.

*Causes Of Dissociated Sensory Loss (usually indicates spinal cord disease but may occur with peripheral neuropathy):*

Spinothalamic (pain and temperature) loss only:

1. Syringomyelia ('cape' distribution).
2. Brown-Séquard syndrome (contralateral leg).
3. Anterior spinal artery thrombosis.
4. Lateral medullary syndrome (contralateral to the other signs).
5. Peripheral neuropathy, e.g., diabetes mellitus, amyloid, Fabry's disease.

Dorsal column (vibration and proprioception) loss only:

1. Subacute combined degeneration.
2. Brown-Séquard syndrome (ipsilateral leg).
3. Spinocerebellar degeneration (e.g., Friedreich's ataxia).
4. Multiple sclerosis.
5. Tabes dorsalis.
6. Sensory neuropathy, e.g., carcinoma.
7. Peripheral neuropathy from diabetes mellitus or hypothyroidism.

*Syringomyelia (A Central Cavity In The Spinal Cord)*
Clinical triad:

1. Loss of pain and temperature over the neck, shoulders and arms ('cape' distribution).

2. Amyotrophy (weakness, atrophy and areflexia) of the arms.
3. Upper motor neurone signs in the lower limbs.
   N.B. There may also be thoracic scoliosis due to asymmetrical weakness of
paravertebral muscles.

## An Approach to Myopathy

### Causes Of Proximal Muscle Weakness

1. Myopathic (qv).
2. Neuromuscular junction disorder, e.g., myaesthenia gravis (p. 124).
3. Neurogenic, e.g., Kugelberg-Welander disease (proximal muscle wasting and
   fasciculation due to anterior horn cell damage—autosomal recessive), motor
   neurone disease, polyradiculopathy.

### Causes Of Myopathy

1. Hereditary muscular dystrophy (qv).
2. Congenital myopathies (rare).
3. Acquired (Mnemonic PACE, PODS):
   (a) Polymyositis or dermatomyositis.
   (b) Alcohol.
   (c) Carcinoma.
   (d) Endocrine, e.g., hypothyroidism, hyperthyroidism, Cushing's syndrome,
       acromegaly, hypopituitarism.
   (e) Periodic paralysis (hyperkalaemic or hypokalaemic or normokalaemic).
   (f) Osteomalacia.
   (g) Drugs, e.g., clofibrate, chloroquine, steroids.
   (h) Sarcoidosis.
       N.B. Causes of proximal myopathy and a peripheral neuropathy include:
   (a) Paraneoplastic syndrome.
   (b) Alcohol.
   (c) Connective tissue disease.

Muscular Dystrophies

1. Duchenne's (pseudohypertrophic) (sex-linked recessive disorder).
   (a) Affects only males (or females with Turner's syndrome).
   (b) The calves and deltoids are hypertrophied early and weak later.
   (c) Early proximal weakness.
   (d) Tendon reflexes are preserved in proportion to muscle strength.
   (e) Severe progressive kyphoscoliosis.
   (f) Heart disease (dilated cardiomyopathy).
   (g) Creatinine kinase level markedly elevated.
   (h) Patients die in the second decade, usually from heart disease.
2. Becker (sex-linked recessive disorder). Same features as Duchenne's but less
   severe, has a later onset and is less rapidly progressive.
3. Limb girdle (autosomal recessive).
   (a) Shoulder or pelvic girdle affected (onset third decade).
   (b) Face and heart usually spared.

**Table 8-45.**   *Causes of Myotonia (all autosomal dominant)*

1. Dystrophia myotonica.
2. Myotonia congenita (myotonia of the tongue and thenar eminence; the recessive form is more severe).
3. Paramyotonia congenita (episodic myotonia after cold exposure).

N.B. Drugs (e.g., clofibrate) can also cause myotonia.

4. Facioscapulohumeral (autosomal dominant).
   (a) Facial and pectoral girdle weakness with hypertrophy of the deltoids (normal pelvic muscles early).
5. Distal dystrophies.
   (a) Autosomal dominant disease which is rare and causes distal muscle atrophy and weakness.
   (b) Dystrophia myotonica (autosomal dominant).

Tests for Myopathy:

1. Creatinine kinase (highest in Duchenne's).
2. Electromyogram.
3. Electrocardiogram (particularly Duchenne's and dystrophia myotonica).
4. Muscle biopsy.

# Dystrophia Myotonica

This patient has noticed some arm weakness. Please examine.

## *Method*

Stand back and you fortunately notice the features of myotonic dystrophy. Proceed as follows.

Observe the face for frontal baldness (the patient may be wearing a wig), dull triangular facies ('hatchet' face), temporalis, masseter and sternomastoid atrophy and partial ptosis. Notice thick spectacles, as these patients develop cataracts, and fine subcapsular deposits which are virtually diagnostic.

Look at the neck for sternomastoid atrophy, then test neck flexion (neck flexion is weak while extension is normal).

Go to the upper limbs. Shake hands (for grip myotonia) and test percussion myotonia. Tapping over the thenar eminence causes contraction then slow relaxation of abductor pollicis brevis (Table 8-45).

Examine the arm now for signs of wasting and weakness, especially of the forearm muscles. Sensory changes from the associated peripheral neuropathy are usually very mild.

Go to the chest and inspect for gynaecomastia.

Next palpate the testes for atrophy.

Examine the lower limbs if there is time. Always ask to test the urine for sugar (diabetes mellitus is commoner in this disease) and ask to examine the cardio-vascular system for cardiomyopathy. Finally test mental status (mild mental retardation is usual).

N.B. Remember the classical EMG finding in dystrophia myotonica of a 'dive bomber' effect with the needle in the muscle at rest.

# Gait

Please examine this patient's gait.

## *Method* (Figure 38)
Make sure the patient's legs are clearly visible. Ask her to hop out of bed (look carefully whilst she is doing so for focal disease), watch her walk normally for a few metres, and then ask her to turn around quickly and walk back towards you.

Next ask her to walk heel-to-toe to exclude a midline cerebellar lesion.

Ask her then to walk on her toes (an S1 lesion will make this impossible) and then on her heels (an L4 or L5 lesion causing foot drop will make this impossible).

Test for proximal myopathy by asking the patient to squat than stand up or sit in a chair and then stand.

Look for Romberg's sign (posterior column loss causes inability to stand stead-ily when the feet are together with the eyes closed, while cerebellar disease causes difficulty when the eyes are open too). Go on and examine the lower limbs depending on your findings.

The typical gaits to recognize are listed in Table 8-46.

# Cerebellum

This patient has noticed a problem with coordination. Please examine.

## *Method*
This patient is likely to have a cerebellar problem (Table 8-47). The only other likely possibilities are posterior column loss or extrapyramidal disease.

Proceed as follows for assessment of cerebellar disease.

Look first for nystagmus, usually jerky horizontal nystagmus with an increased amplitude on looking towards the side of the lesion.

Assess speech next. Ask the patient to say 'British Constitution' and 'West Register Street'. Cerebellar speech is jerky, explosive and loud, with irregular separation of syllables.

Go to the upper limbs. Ask the patient to extend his arms and look for arm drift and static tremor due to hypotonia of the agonist muscles. Test tone. Hypotonia is due to loss of a facilitatory influence on the spinal motor neurones.

Next perform the finger-nose-test—the patient touches his nose, then rotates his finger and touches your finger. Note any intention tremor (tremor increasing as the

**Figure 38.**  *Gait*

Standing (legs fully exposed)

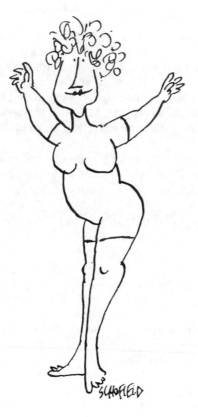

GENERAL INSPECTION
  Deformity
  Diagnostic facies (Table 8-29)
  Upper limb lesions
  Focal neurological disease, e.g., wasting
  Fasciculation
  Abnormal movements
ASK THE PATIENT TO:
  Walk normally and turn around
    quickly (abnormal gait)
  Heel-toe walking (cerebellar disease)
  Walk on toes (S1)
  Walk on heels (L4 or L5)
  Squat (proximal myopathy)
  Romberg's sign—feet together with:
    Eyes closed (posterior columns)
    Eyes open (cerebellar disease)

EXAMINE LOWER LIMBS (p. 230)

**Table 8-46.**  *Typical Gaits*

1. Hemiparetic. The foot is plantar flexed and the leg is swung in a lateral arc.
2. Paraparetic (scissor gait).
3. Extrapyramidal (e.g., Parkinson's disease)
   a) hesitation in starting
   b) shuffling
   c) freezing
   d) festination (the patient hurries forward trying to catch up with his or her centre of gravity)
   e) propulsion (push the patient gently—he or she will be unable to stop), retropulsion.
4. Cerebellar (a drunken gait which is wide based or reeling on a narrow base; the patient staggers towards the affected side).
5. Apraxic (prefrontal lobe) (feet appear glued to floor when erect, but move more easily when the patient is supine).
6. Posterior column lesion (clumsy slapping down of the feet on a broad base).
7. Distal weakness (high-stepping gait).
8. Proximal weakness (a waddling gait).

**Table 8-47.**  *Causes of Cerebellar Disease*

**Unilateral**
1. Space-occupying lesion (tumour, abscess, granuloma)
2. Ischaemia (vertebrobasilar disease)
3. Paraneoplastic syndrome
4. Multiple sclerosis
5. Trauma

**Bilateral**
1. Drugs, e.g, phenytoin
2. Friedreich's ataxia
3. Hypothyroidism
4. Paraneoplastic syndrome
5. Multiple sclerosis
6. Trauma ('punch drunk')
7. Arnold-Chiari malformation
8. Alcohol
9. Large space-occupying lesion, cerebrovascular disease, rare metabolic diseases

**Midline**
1. Paraneoplastic syndrome
2. Midline tumour

**Rostral Vermis lesion (only lower limbs affected)**
1. Alcohol (commonest cause of a cerebellar lesion in Australia)

**Table 8-48.** *Clinical Features of Friedreich's Ataxia (autosomal recessive)*

*Usually a young person with:*

1. Cerebellar signs (bilateral) including nystagmus
2. Posterior column loss in the limbs
3. Upper motor neurone signs in the limbs (although ankle reflexes are absent)
4. Peripheral neuropathy
5. Optic atrophy
6. Pes cavus, cocking of the toes, kyphoscoliosis
7. Cardiomyopathy (ECG abnormalities occur in more than 50% of cases)
8. Diabetes mellitus
9. Normal mentation

target is approached due to loss of cerebellar connections in the brainstem) and past pointing (the patient overshooting the target).

Test rapid alternating movements; the patient taps alternately the palm and back of one hand on his other hand or thigh. Inability to perform this movement smoothly is called dysdiadochokinesis.

Test rebound—ask the patient to lift his arms quickly from the sides then stop. Hypotonia causes the patient to be unable to stop his arms.

Always demonstrate each movement for the patient's benefit, asking him to copy you.

Go on to examine the legs. Again test tone here. Then perform the heel-shin test, looking for accuracy of fine movement when the patient slides his heel down the shin slowly on each side for several cycles. Next ask him to lift his big toe up to touch your finger, looking for intention tremor. Ask the patient then to tap each foot rapidly on a firm surface.

Look for truncal ataxia by asking the patient to fold his arms and sit up. While he is sitting, ask him to put his legs over the side of the bed and test for pendular knee jerks.

Test gait (the patient will stagger towards the affected side).

If there is time look for possible causes of the problem. If there is an obvious unilateral lesion, auscultate over the cerebellum, then proceed to the cranial nerves and look for evidence of a cerebellopontine angle tumour (V, VII, VIII nerves affected) (p. 218) and the lateral medullary syndrome (p. 209). Always look in the fundi for papilloedema. Next examine for peripheral evidence of malignant disease and vascular disease (carotid bruits).

If there is a midline lesion only (i.e., truncal ataxia or abnormal heel-toe walking or abnormal speech), consider either a midline tumour or a paraneoplastic syndrome. If there is bilateral disease, look for signs of multiple sclerosis (p. 122), Friedreich's ataxia (pes cavus being the most helpful initial clue) (Tables 8-48 and 8-49), and hypothyroidism (rare). Alcoholic cerebellar degeneration (which affects the anterior lobe of the cerebellar vermis) classically spares the arms.

If there are, in addition, upper motor neurone signs, consider the causes in Table 8-50.

**Table 8-49.**  *Causes of Pes Cavus*

1. Friedreich's ataxia or other spinocerebellar degenerations
2. Hereditary motor and sensory neuropathy (HMSN)
3. Neuropathies in childhood

**Table 8-50.**  *Causes of Spastic and Ataxic Paraparesis (upper motor neurone and cerebellar signs combined)*

*In adolescence:*
1. Spinocerebellar degeneration, e.g., Marie's spastic ataxia

*In young adults:*
1. Multiple sclerosis (p. 122)
2. Syphilitic meningomyelitis
3. Spinocerebellar degeneration
4. Arnold-Chiari malformation or other lesions at the craniospinal junction

*In later life:*
1. Multiple sclerosis
2. Syringomyelia
3. Infarction (in upper pons or internal capsule—'ataxic hemiparesis')
4. Lesion at the craniospinal junction, e.g., meningioma

Don't forget common unrelated diseases (e.g., cervical spondylosis and cerebellar degeneration from alcohol) may occur together by chance.

# Parkinson's Disease

This patient has Parkinson's disease. Please assess.

## *Method*

Look at the patient first. Note the obvious lack of facial expression ('mask-like') and paucity of movement.

Ask the patient to walk, turn quickly, and stop and restart. Particularly note difficulty starting, shuffling, freezing and festination. It is probably a little dangerous to look for propulsion or retropropulsion (Table 8-46).

Ask the patient to return to bed and look for a resting tremor with the arms relaxed (Table 8-51). The characteristic movement is described as pill rolling. On finger-nose testing, a resting tremor diminishes, but action tremor may appear. Test wrist tone, feeling for cog-wheel or lead pipe rigidity. Reinforce this by asking him to turn his head from side to side. Test for abnormal rapid alternating movements. Look also for involuntary movements produced by medication use.

Go to the face. Note titubation (tremor), absence of blinking, dribbling of saliva and lack of expression. Test the glabellar tap; the sign is positive when the patient continues to blink after the middle finger taps several times over the glabella from behind—it is important that your finger is out of his line of vision. Test speech then, which is typically monotonous, soft, poorly articulated and faint. Look at the

**Table 8-51.** *A Classification of Tremor*

1. Parkinsonian (4 to 6 Hertz)—resting tremor.
2. Action tremor. Present throughout movement but resolves at rest:
   a) thyrotoxicosis
   b) anxiety
   c) drugs
   d) familial
   e) idiopathic (most common).
3. Intention tremor (cerebellar disease). Increases towards the target.
4. Midbrain ('red nucleus') tremor—abduction-adduction movements of upper limbs with flexion-extension of wrists (usually associated with intention tremor).

N.B. Flapping (asterixis) is not strictly a tremor but a sudden brief loss of tone in hepatic failure (p. 75), cardiac failure (p. 38), respiratory failure (p. 50), or renal failure (p. 113).

ocular movements for supranuclear gaze palsies (p. 217). Feel for a greasy or sweaty brow (due to autonomic dysfunction).

Ask the patient to write (looking for micrographia), and test the frontal lobe reflexes and higher centres (looking for evidence of dementia).

Causes of Parkinsonism:

1. Idiopathic (Parkinson's disease).
2. Drugs, e.g., phenothiazines, methyldopa.
3. Postencephalitis.
4. Other, e.g., toxins (carbon monoxide, manganese), Wilson's disease, Steele-Richardson syndrome, Shy-Drager syndrome, syphilis, tumour.
   N.B. Atherosclerosis is a controversial cause of Parkinsonism.

## Chorea

Examine this patient's arms.

### Method

Happily you notice an extrapyramidal choreiform movement disorder. Choreiform movements are non-repetitive, abrupt, involuntary, more distal jerky movements, which the patient often attempts to disguise by completing the involuntary movement with a voluntary one. This is due to a lesion of the corpus striatum. HEMIBALLISMUS is unilateral and usually involves rotary movements of proximal joints. This is caused by a subthalamic nucleus lesion on the opposite side. ATHETOSIS involves slow, sinuous distal writhing movements at rest. This is due to a lesion of the outer segment of the putamen.

If the patient has chorea, proceed as follows.

First shake the patient's hand, for a lack of sustained grip ('milkmaid grip'). Ask the patient to hold his hands out and look for a choreic posture (finger and thumb hyperextension and wrist flexion due to hypotonia). Note any signs of vasculitis. Go to the face and look at the eyes for exophthalmos, Kayser-Fleischer

**Table 8-52.** *Causes of Chorea*

1. Huntington's disease (autosomal dominant)
2. Sydenham's chorea (rheumatic fever)
3. Senility
4. Wilson's disease
5. Drugs, e.g., phenothiazines, the contraceptive pill, phenytoin, L-dopa
6. Vasculitis or connective tissue disease, e.g., systemic lupus erythematosus (p. 97)
7. Thyrotoxicosis (very rare) (p. 187)
8. Polycythaemia or other causes of hyperviscosity (very rare) (p. 82)
9. Viral encephalitis (very rare)

rings and conjunctival injection. Ask the patient to poke his tongue out and note a serpentine tongue (moving in and out). Notice any rash (e.g., lupus).

If the patient is young, examine the heart, for signs of rheumatic fever.

Test the knee jerks (pendular) and the higher centres (for Huntington's disease). The causes are summarized in Table 8-52.

# FURTHER READING

*You will find it very good practice always to verify your references, sir.*

*Martin Ruth (1755–1854)*

Candidates for the examination must read widely. This particularly applies to the postgraduate candidate who wishes to pass both the written and oral tests. It is very important to spend plenty of time on your weak areas where you have had the least clinical experience.

We have listed below some of the texts which may be useful to candidates. Each section is divided into two parts where applicable. Concise textbooks refer to books which are particularly useful to undergradutes, but do have some relevant material for postgraduate students of internal medicine. Specialist textbooks refer to texts which are of particular relevance to postgraduates, although undergraduates may also find these useful. For further suggestions, see the recommendations from the American College of Physicians entitled 'A Library for Internists' published every three years in *Annals of Internal Medicine*. Although it is unlikely that even the hardest working candidates will read all these books, we believe reference to some of them will be invaluable.

## GENERAL TEXTS

### Concise Textbooks

Rubenstein D, Wayne D. Lecture notes on clinical medicine. 3rd ed. Oxford: Blackwell, 1985. (Outlines clearly and concisely the clinical approach.)

### Specialist Textbooks

Wilson JD, Petersdorf RG, Adams RD, et al (ed). Harrison's principles of internal medicine. 12th ed. New York: McGraw Hill, 1990.
Wilson JD, Petersdorf RG, Adams RD, et al (eds). Harrison's principles of internal medicine. 12th ed. Pretest self-assessment and review. New York: McGraw Hill, 1991.

Weatherall DJ, Ledingham JGG, Ward DA (eds). Oxford textbook of medicine. 2nd ed. Oxford University Press, 1987.

American College of Physicians. Medical knowledge self assessment program IX, 1991.

Talley NJ. Internal medicine: the essential facts. Sydney: MacLennan and Petty, 1990.

# AIDS TO PHYSICAL EXAMINATION

## Concise Textbooks

Talley NJ, O'Connor S. Clinical examination. A guide to physical diagnosis. 2nd ed. Sydney: MacLennan and Petty, 1991.

Scheil MC, Tiller DL, Walsh JC, Furkin FC. A system of signs. 4th ed. ANZ. Book Co., 1982.

Zatouroff M. A colour atlas of physical signs in general medicine. London: Wolfe, 1976.

Schneiderman H. Bedside diagnosis. An annotated bibliography of recent literature on interviewing and physical examination. American College of Physicians, 1988.

# SUBSPECIALITY TEXTS

## Cardiology

### Concise Textbooks

Julian DG. Cardiology. 5th ed. London: Balliére Tindall, 1988.

Sokolow M, McIlroy MB, Cheitlin MD. Clinical cardiology. 5th ed. Norwalk: Appleton Lange, 1989.

Schamroth L. An introduction to electrocardiography. 6th ed. Oxford: Blackwell, 1983.

### Specialist Textbooks

Braunwald E (ed). Heart disease: A textbook of cardiovascular medicine. 3rd ed. Philadelphia: Saunders, 1988. (N.B. Read particularly chapters 1, 2 and 6.)

Giuliani ER. (ed.). Cardiology: Fundamentals and practise. 2nd ed. Chicago: Mosby Year Book, 1990 (a very comprehensive up-to-date reference).

## Respiratory

### Concise Textbooks

Campbell IA, Schonell M. Respiratory medicine. 2nd ed. Edinburgh: Churchill Livingstone, 1984. (N.B. A very good introductory textbook.)

Brewis RAL. Lecture notes on respiratory disease. 3rd ed. Oxford: Blackwell, 1985.

### Specialist Textbooks

West JB. Pulmonary pathophysiology: the essentials. 3rd ed. Baltimore, London: Williams & Wilkins, 1987.

Seaton A, Seaton D, Leitch AG. Crofton and Douglas's respiratory diseases. 4th ed. Oxford: Blackwell Scientific, 1989. (Superb!)

## Gastroenterology and Liver Disease

### Concise Textbook

Powell L, Piper D. Fundamentals of gastroenterology. 5th ed. Sydney: McGraw-Hill 1990. (N.B. A good introductory undergraduate textbook on this subject.)

### Specialist Textbooks

Sleisenger MH, Fordtran JS. (eds) Gastrointestinal disease. 4th ed. Philadelphia: WB Saunders, 1988.

Sherlock S. Diseases of the liver and biliary system. 8th ed. Oxford: Blackwell, 1989.

## Haematology

### Concise Textbooks

Waterbury L. Hematology for the house officer. 3rd ed. Baltimore: Williams and Wilkins, 1988.

Rappaport SI. Introduction to hematology. 2nd ed. Philadelphia: Lippincott, 1987.

### Specialist Textbook

Jandl J. Blood: A textbook of hematology. Boston: Little Brown, 1987. (N.B. A detailed reference source.)

## Rheumatology and Immunology

### Concise Textbooks

Mason M, Currey HLF. Introduction to clinical rheumatology. 3rd ed. London: Pitman, 1986.

Edmonds J, Hughes G. Lecture notes on rheumatology. Oxford: Blackwell, 1986.

### Specialist Textbooks

Primer on the rheumatic diseases. 8th ed. Atlanta, Georgia: Arthritis Foundation, 1983.

Hughes GRV. Connective tissue diseases. 3rd ed. Oxford: Blackwell, 1987.

Stites DP, Stolo JD, Fudenberg HH, Wells JV. Basic and clinical immunology. 6th ed. Los Altos, California: Lange, 1987.

Roitt I, Brostoff J, Male DK. Immunology. St. Louis: Mosby, 1985. (Excellent summary with very clear illustrations).

# Neurology

## Concise Textbooks

McLeod JG, Lance JW. Introductory neurology. Melbourne: Blackwell, 1986. (N.B. A clear, concise textbook.)

Weiner HL, Levitt LP. Neurology for the house officer. 4th ed. Baltimore, London: Williams & Wilkins, 1989. (N.B. A practical approach to neurology is succinctly outlined, making this a very valuable book.)

Bickerstaff ER, Spillane JA. Neurological examination in clinical practice. 5th ed. Oxford: Blackwell, 1989. (N.B. Highly recommended.)

## Specialist Textbooks

Walton JN. Brain's diseases of the nervous system. 9th ed. Oxford: University Press, 1985.

Montgomery EB, Wall M, Henderson VW. Principles of neurologic diagnosis. Little Brown and Company, 1986. (N.B. an excellent instruction guide that uses cases to teach diagnosis.)

Medical Research Council. Memorandum No. 45. Aids to examination of the peripheral nervous system. London: Her Majesty's Stationery Office, 1976. (N.B. Very clear photographs and illustrations make this an invaluable reference book.)

Patten J. Neurological differential diagnoses—an illustrated approach. London: Harold Starke, 1977. (N.B. Refer to this book for the clear, useful illustrations.)

# Renal Disease

## Concise Textbooks

Brenner B, Coe FL, Rector FC. Clinical nephrology. Philadelphia: WB Saunders, 1987.

Abuelo JG. Renal pathophysiology—the essentials. Baltimore: Williams and Wilkins, 1989. (N.B. Includes clinically orientated problems with solutions.)

## Specialist Textbook

Schrier RW (ed). Renal and electrolyte disorders. 3rd ed. Boston: Little, Brown, 1986. (N.B. Although difficult reading, well worthwhile as some multiple choice questions have been taken from its contents.)

# Endocrinology

## Concise Textbooks

Larkins RG. A practical approach to endocrine disorders. Sydney: Williams and Wilkins, 1985.

Greenspan FS, Forsham PH (eds). Basic and clinical endocrinology. 2nd ed. Los Altos: Lange Medical; sydeny: Ramsay, 1986.

Beigelman PM, Kumar D. Diabetes mellitus for the house officer. Baltimore: Williams and Wilkins, 1986.

## Specialist Textbooks

Kohler PO, Jordan RM. Clinical endocrinology. New York: John Wiley and Sons, 1986. (Emphasises clinical aspects.)

DeGroot LJ (ed). Endocrinology. 2nd ed. Philadelphia: WB Saunders, 1989.

# Dermatology

### Concise Textbooks

Lynch PJ. Dermatology for the house officer. 2nd ed. Baltimore: Williams and Wilkins, 1986.

Fitzpatrick TB, Polano MK, Suurmond D. Colour atlas and synopsis of clinical dermatology. New York: McGraw-Hill, 1983.

# Pharmacology

### Concise Textbooks

Katzung BG. Basic and clinical pharmacology. 5th ed. Norwalk: Appleton and Lange, 1991.

### Specialist Textbook

Gilman AG, et al (ed). Goodman and Gilman's the pharmacological basis of therapeutics. 8th ed. New York: Pergamon, 1990 (Still the leading text.)

# Radiology

### Concise Textbook

Squire LF, Novelline RA. Fundamentals of radiology. 4th ed. Cambridge: Harvard University Press, 1988. (An excellent introduction and highly recommended.)

### Specialist Textbook

Lillington GA. A diagnostic approach to chest diseases. Differential diagnosis based on roentgenographic patterns. 3rd ed. Baltimore: Williams and Wilkins, 1987.

# Infectious Diseases

### Concise Textbook

Emond RTD, Rowland HAK. A colour atlas of infectious diseases. 2nd ed. London: Wolfe Medical, 1987.

### Specialist Textbook

Christie AB (ed.) Infectious diseases: Epidemiology and clinical practise of diseases. 4th ed. New York: Churchill Livingstone, 1987. (A comprehensive reference book.)

# JOURNALS

All postgraduate candidates must read the journals because textbooks are always somewhat out of date by the time they are published.

The following journals are specifically recommended by the Royal Australasian College of Physicians:

1. *New England Journal of Medicine*
2. *Lancet*
3. *Annals of Internal Medicine*
4. *British Medical Journal*
5. *American Journal of Medicine*
6. *Australian and New Zealand Journal of Medicine*

N.B. The excellent review articles and editorials should be studied. Topics often crop up from these articles, particularly those published in the 3 years or so prior to the multiple-choice questions being set.

# Index

*Entries in italics refer to X-ray illustrations.*

## A

abdominal examination  165, 178–81
abdominal masses, causes of  180
  *see also* kidneys; liver; spleen
abdominal X-ray  70, 118
accommodation reflex  212
acetylcholine receptor test  125
acid-base disturbances  20
acromegaly  192, 194–5, 196
Addison's disease  195, 197
adrenal cortex  19
adrenal medulla  19
alcohol
  and triglyceridaemia  42
alpha-1 antitrypsin deficiency  56
  in liver disease  74
anaemia  13
analgesic nephropathy  113
Angioid streaks  196
angiotensin-converting enzyme  60–1
ankle  232
ankylosing spondylitis, X-ray changes
  206
anorexia nervosa  15, 20
anosmia  211
anterior pituitary lobe  19
anti-nRNP  99
antibiotics  17, 22
  and infective endocarditis  35
  *see also* drugs
anticholinesterase  125
antithymocyte globulin  46
antitumour drugs  18
antiviral agents  22
aortic incompetence  145–6
  in infective endocarditis  35

aortic stenosis  146
  in infective endocarditis  35
apex beat  138
aphasia  225
Argyll Robertson pupil  213
Arnold Chiari malformation  221
arrythmias  10
arterial blood gases
  in bronchiectasis  50
  in COPD  55
  and lung fibrosis  57
  in polycythaemia  86
  in pulmonary fibrosis  57
arterial pulse character  138
arthritis, in sarcoidosis  59, 60
asbestos lung disease  57
ascites  75
  percussion in  179, 181
  treatment  77
  *see also* liver disease
ascitic tap  74, 75, 76
asthma  11, 55
atrial natiuretic factor  19
atrial septal defect (ASD)  142, *150*, 154
atrial septal defect, secundum type  36
auscultation  139
  for respiratory disease  162, 164
autoimmune-associated disease  196
azathioprine  46, 101
  in kidney transplant  122

## B

$B_{12}$ absorption  66
$B_{12}$ binding capacity
  in polycythaemia  86

*Hos successus aliit; possunt, quia posse videntur.*
*Success nourished them; they seemed to be able, and so they were able.*

Virgil (70-19 B.C.)


GOOD LUCK!

Tue

Wed

Thu

Fri

Sat

Sun

Mon

Tue

Wed

Thu

---

Data

Literature

X-Rays

ECgs

Long cases

Ryder

Emergencies

Background
    knowlege